The Muse in the Bottle

The Muse in the Bottle

GREAT WRITERS ON THE JOYS OF DRINKING

Edited by

Charles A. Coulombe

CITADEL PRESS
Kensington Publishing Corp.
www.kensingtonbooks.com

CITADEL PRESS BOOKS are published by

Kensington Publishing Corp.
850 Third Avenue
New York, NY 10022

First Printing: July 2002

10 9 8 7 6 5 4 3 2 1

Printed in the United States of America

Library of Congress Control Number: 2002100668

ISBN 0-8065-2371-9

Dedication
to
Guy Joseph Conrad Coulombe
(1926–1996)
My beloved father, who taught me both how to drink and to be a man
and
to
Jess Harrahill
Once and future drinking companion, and current defender of our freedoms

This book is fondly dedicated, in memory of good times past and
hope of future ones to come.

CONTENTS

ACKNOWLEDGMENTS

I *would like to thank, first, Jake Elwell, my agent; Richard Ember, my editor; Bruce Bender at Kensington; Stephen Lemons for rallying support at the last; and Nicholas Lanier and Phillip Coulombe, for typing everything into the computer.*

My personal gratitude must further be extended, in a book like this, to those with whom I have most enjoyed sharing libations. In the gallery of the deceased, one looks first to my father, Guy Coulombe; to Charl Van Horn; Paul Edwin Zimmer; thence to Henry Brandon, Virginia O'Brien, George Diestel, Hugh Beaumont, Frank Faylen, and the other irreplaceables of the late lamented Masquers' Club.

Among the living: Duncan Anderson, Dr. Albert Audet, William Biersach III, Joanna and James Bogle, Richard Bost, Ryan Brookhart, Bonnie and Tim Callahan, Andre N. Coulombe, Silvana, Richard, and Joseph Cowden-Guido, Corey Crouch, Matthew Crow, J. Fred Farrell, Jr., Brian Feeney, Tim Feeney, Stephen Frankini, Jane Gartenmann, Matthew S. Hale, Eve and Brian Hansen, Jess Harrahill, Christian Hasse, Stephan, Baron von Hoeller-Bertram, Stephen Kearney, Scott Keller, Gilles, Comte de Kerangal, Nicholas, George, Alexei, and Pierre, Barons von Knupffer, David Lumsden of Cushnie, Tequila Mockingbird, Anthony, Benjamin, and Geoffrey Mull, Christiane and Axel Mullers, John O'Malley, Albert Petho, Gary Potter, John Prizer, Judith Richardson, Dominic Rouvier, Katherine and Charles Shepphard, Sasha Suscenko, Dag Syversen, Jim Thomas, Laurel Tropp, Roberta "Chantal" Tropp, Jay Weiner, John Zmirak, and an ever-expanding cast.

INTRODUCTION

Was there ever a more sublime act outside of religion than drinking alcohol? Whether you speak of banquets or taverns, weddings or wakes, get-togethers with friends or romantic evenings for two, the juice of the grain or the grape always adds to the occasion its own special alchemy. Consecrated by both tradition and experience, imbibing of spirits is one of the most universal acts of humanity.

Not surprisingly, it has been immortalized in song and story. Prohibitionists, moral "reformers," and the various victims of alcohol abuse notwithstanding, from the earliest days of writing—in Egypt, Palestine, Greece, and Rome—to the present, prose writers and poets alike have written in praise of drinking and the festivity that attends it. Because of the wide range of activities involved with the practice, writers on drinking have touched virtually every aspect of the human experience: birth, death, loss, love, camaraderie, hunting, and traveling. Most, including this present editor, would agree with the late Brendan Behan's observation, "I'm a drinker with a writing problem."

Perhaps the glow of good-feeling that can result from the well-downed drink is summed up best in the description of the mythical "Old Mr. Boston," which opens the 1935 edition of the famous bartender's guide put out by the distillery of the same name. Below the picture of a portly Dickensian figure in top hat are the words: "Sirs:—May we now present to you Old Mr. Boston in permanent form. We know you are going to like him. He is a jolly fellow, one of those rare individuals, everlastingly young, a distinct personality and famous throughout the land for his sterling qualities and genuine good fellowship. His friends number in the millions those who are great and those who are near great even as you and I. He is joyful and ever ready to accept the difficult role of 'Life of the Party,' a sympathetic friend who may be relied upon in any emergency . . . Follow his advice and there will be many good times in store for you. Gentlemen, Old Mr. Boston."

It is this feeling of geniality, of excitement, of contentedness, and of sheer joy, which the best of writing about drinking evokes; but like the real thing, it sometimes also forces an encounter with truth. As my friend and drinking companion Nicholas von Knupffer has well quoted:

> Not drunk is he who from the floor,
> Can rise again and drink some more.
>
> But drunk is he who prostrate lies,
> Without the power to drink nor rise.

As renowned as the act are the favored snug harbors wherein it often takes place. From the taverns of Greece and Rome to the late and unlamented fern bars of the early 1980s, such locales—whether in fiction or reality—have often provided refuge from life's pains, and tastes of the amicability and unity which, in a perfect world, would reign supreme. One female witness in the old *Perry Mason* television show, asked by that star defense attorney why she spent four hours in a watering hole, replied: "After a few drinks, a bar becomes a fairy land; the people there are so courteous . . . and considerate." Often they particularly seem that way if they tolerate one's behavior after the seventh round.

Nevertheless, contemplating my favorite places, from elevated bars like the American Bar at London's Savoy Hotel, to dives on the order of the Frolic Room on Hollywood Boulevard, they do have that one element in common—they provide *sanctuary*. So often, the folk one meets in these places appear—at least for the moment—to share one's views, one's hopes, and one's fears. The ultimate time for gleaning barroom wisdom seems to be about four in the afternoon. Only truly dedicated drinkers, who really have nothing better to do with their time, will be found then.

In times of disaster, such as the nation experienced on September 11, 2001 (or as we Californians do after every major quake), the bars fill. Modern-day prohibitionists are always displeased by such "unhealthy" behavior. But wiser heads realize that in the face of horror, humanity has a need to reach for the familiar and the communal: comfort food, old bars, and good booze.

The best bars will, later in the day, offer a mix of such grizzled veterans with younger apprentice types. In healthier cultures, such as in Europe, whole families may be found in local pubs: adolescents learning from their elders the fine art of drinking. Certainly, the longing for community is to some degree fulfilled in the most successful gin mills. This is a longing that grows ever keener as modern technology further isolates individuals.

A word ought to be offered for the bars of private clubs. During the 1980s, when I was a young man, fortune brought me to the venerable Masquers' Club, at 1765 N. Sycamore, in Hollywood. Founded as the West Coast affiliate of the still more aged Lambs' Club in New York, the Masquers' was, like its parent, an actor's club. In my day, many an old character actor haunted its storied bar, modeled after one in Stratford on Avon, and used as "Clay's Grill" during the final 1965–1966 season of *Perry Mason.* Most of the haunters were living, but Alan Mowbray, deceased since 1967, made more than a few appearances. Strange tales emanated from the bar, and became stranger as the night and the drinks progressed. When a member died (a not uncommon occurrence), his favorite drink was set up for a day in his memory.

Alas, as my friend Stephen Frankini has observed, "All good things must go." So it was with the Masquers'. But the bar itself was removed successively to the Variety Arts Club, downtown, and at last to the Mayflower Club in North Hollywood, where it resides at present. Mentioning to a group of cronies one Thanksgiving that "they saved the Masquers' Bar," one of them (who had shared a few adventures there) shot back, "from the people who brought you, 'They Saved Hitler's Brain.'" Such is the affection such a place can instill even in occasional guests.

So it is with the Lansdowne Club in London, much resorted to by many of my friends there. One in particular, Alexander Suscenko, is famed for his practice of, after having reached a certain point of inebriation, saying, "It's all very confusing. I'm confused. Are you confused? It's all terribly confusing." This is about all to be extracted from him for the rest of the evening. Rather than being tiresome, it is a refreshing acceptance of reality in a world filled with self-proclaimed experts.

With the bar as meat rack or trysting place for alternative lifestyles, I have as little to do in this anthology as in real life. But it must be admitted that an alcoholic haze often lends romance to an evening and beauty to a face. As the late Morey Amsterdam observed, "A woman looks her best ten minutes before last call." Alas, such beauty, like the gold of the fairies, is often fleeting and vanishes at daybreak.

In tribute to the love your author holds for so many of these refuges, after certain selections is a brief comment by an employee of one or another of my favorite taverns.

For many of us, drinking is a rite of passage. By it we show that we have left the supervision of our parents behind with our childhood. Of course, we often mark this passage with behavior that would have been childish on the playground; but never mind. College and university annals the world over are replete with legendary deeds performed by students under the influence. One Cambridge college boasts of an automobile disassembled and lovingly rebuilt on a roof by a jolly band of collegiate inebriates, and many are the audacious thefts and/or returns of large and inappropriate objects performed under similar circumstances. Memory reminds me of a Catholic Harvard man who, after a convivial evening at Jake Wirth's, climbed the 18 or so foot-high statue of Unitarian shaman William Ellery Channing in Boston's Public Garden. Having imbibed deeply, the student was able to bestow upon that historic figure the Baptism denied him by Unitarian dogma.

So it was in my time; after two years at New Mexico Military Institute, a military junior college where such escapades had to be pursued with utmost caution, lest expulsion follow, this writer landed at a civilian college. Joining a fraternity, he soon found himself engaged in similar goings-on. Years later, having arrived at a reputation as a serious author and journalist, he was consulted by a young freshman at USD who had become a fan of his work.

"Mr. Coulombe," he telephoned. "It's rush week down here. I was wondering if I should rush a frat."

"Well," I replied, "I was an Omicron Omega [NOT the real name]. They were a blast!"

"I'll try them," said the serious young scholar.

A week later he called, much saddened. "Gee, Mr. Coulombe, they must have changed a lot since your day."

"Why do you say so?"

"Well, they're nothing but a bunch of empty-headed booze hounds!"

"Yes, that's what I remember!"

Disappointed, he did not pledge the OO's. But in time he did find a frat to his liking and indulged in his own liquor-powered zany high jinks. These events remind one of a terrible truth: it is easy to be interesting when young; one must fight increasingly ever after to avoid becoming a bore. Sometimes alcohol helps in this quest—sometimes not.

Another arena in which drink plays a part is the party, feast, or banquet. Whether commemorating a specific event, or just held to be held, these affairs can be the stuff of life, or living death, depending upon host and guests. When successful, cocktails, wine, and champagne serve as rocket fuel, driving wit to giddy heights. But even when the opposite occurs, drinking can usually prevent the boredom from becoming too intense.

Usually, but not always. I remember a party in New Jersey I once attended, the host of which was blessed with an extended family rumored to have mob connections. Whether or not that was true, the quick repartee often found at Italian get-togethers was replaced by an endless tale about nothing, listlessly recited by a large-girthed patriarch. While family members listened in rapt attention, I drank ever deeper of their excellent Scotch. Alas, inebriation eluded me, and I heard the whole thing. It was a long night.

At any rate, a good piece of the drinking experience is to be found within these pages. From the joy of hilarity to the dejection of hangover, it is here. The pieces in this anthology range in time from the Bible and the Graeco-Roman classics to the present, and cover the whole breadth of human celebrative drinking. From Roman banquets to Norse sagas, through eighteenth-century picaresque novels, up to our present day, stories and essays that regale the reader with scenes of joyful libation are served up.

Among some of the better known authors are Irving, Fielding, Dickens, Lovecraft, Fitzgerald, and Thorne Smith. A few selections are published here for the first time. Here you find banquets, weddings, tavern drinking, friendship pledging, hunt parties, toasting, speakeasies, and much else.

These writings chronicle the human experience at its most heightened—when alcohol strips away the dullness of mundane, everyday existence and gilds the ordinary with either illusion or deeper reality. Running over a wide territory in both time and space, they show us that alcohol is one of the most unitive of human experiences: "The Seven Sages of the Bamboo Grove" of the Warring States period in fifth-century China had much in common with the absinthe-swigging nineteenth-century French Symbolists. The revelers of the ancient Roman *Satyricon* were blood (or booze) brothers to the tavern-goers of *Tom Jones*.

One will notice that in American letters, the high point of joyous alcohol writing was the period between the Wars, when Prohibition's demise allowed the toper to breathe freely again. Also, the Celts, legendary for their love of drink, are well represented: Arthur Machen for the Welsh, and a son of the Emerald Isle, Frank McCourt.

Themes run through almost every selection: the chameleon-like, ever-changing nature of the drinking experience; in one night—even in one drink—one's emotions can run the whole gamut, from love to hate to fear. One's dignity dissolves, or is rediscovered; one escapes responsibility, or embraces it. But all with an alcohol-induced intensity. Even the most jovial selections here have a bit of an edge to them; but almost all of the darker ones carry some hint of redemption.

Another point that hit me very strongly in the selection process is that plentiful as booze-prose is, it is far outnumbered by similar poetry. This perhaps is because verse is far easier for most writers under the influence. Nevertheless, despite the oceans of verse available, I have confined myself to a few examples. Should public thirst demand more from me along these lines, I shall dip deeply into the poetic fountain in a subsequent volume.

It will also be noticed by those with an interest in biography that the majority of the gentlemen (and ladies) of the pen are extremely fond of liquor. Gary Potter, the sage of D.C., is of the opinion that this trait (shared, as he points out, most commonly with doctors), arises for the same reason as the thirst of the medicine men; both guilds make life-and-death decisions constantly. Even though the one set deals with flesh and the other with paper, subjectively, the effect is the same.

In alcohol, as in literature, the highest aspirations of Humanity can be made manifest. The eternal yearning of all people everywhere for a joy that transcends the pain and the boredom of life—found nowhere permanently this side of the grave—may, most of the world's cultures have agreed, be glimpsed for short periods through the prism of drink. Thus, even in the Old Testament we are advised to "Give strong drink to them that are sad, and wine to them that are grieved in mind: Let them drink, and forget their want, and remember their sorrow no more" (Prov. 31:6–7). Of Heaven itself, we are told no more than that there is wine there, for Christ says at the Last Supper, "And I say to you: I will not drink from henceforth of this fruit of the vine, until that day, when I shall drink it new with you in the kingdom of my Father" (Matt. 26:29). An image, perhaps, of the ultimate celebration.

In a word, the writings in this collection show drinking as a vehicle for humanity's greatest joys and highest aspirations—a vehicle present in all times, and all places.

Charles A. Coulombe
Arcadia, California
Christmas, 2001

The Muse in the Bottle

Although the following Mexican folktale is a relatively late composition, having arisen after the Spanish conquest in 1521, we have it first because of the events it describes and the truths it imparts—which will be demonstrated throughout the rest of the book.

Wine and the Devil

(from "A Pack Load of Mexican Tales")

The world had been made and God was preparing to plant the vineyard when the devil asked, "What are you doing?"

"I'm planting some grapes," said God. "There will be times in the life of man when he will need wine to cheer him up."

"Would you mind if I help?" asked the devil.

God meditated for a bit. "What is he up to now?" thought He. At last, feeling no harm could be done, He said, "All right, you may help."

"You will be surprised at my efficiency," said the devil.

He went to work immediately. First he killed a mockingbird and sprinkled the blood along the rows. Then he killed a lion, and then a swine, and sprinkled their blood too, from one end of the vineyard to the other.

"A' 'sta listo," said he. "Now we are ready and we shall see what happens."

We are all well aware what happened. When a man first begins drinking he feels the effects of the bird's blood and sings. He continues to drink until fired by the lion's blood; then he fights. His thirst increases until he has drunk as deep as the swine's blood, and the next thing we know he is in the gutter.

Ay, que mala suerte! What ill fate!

 What differentiates Keen's from other bars is that it's a museum of drinking.
—RAUL, BARTENDER, KEEN'S CHOPHOUSE, 72 W. 36TH STREET, NEW YORK

From J. Frank Dobie, ed., *Puro Mexicano* (Texas Folklore Society, vol. XII). Denton: University of North Texas Press, 3rd printing, 1980. © 1935 by Texas Folklore Society. Reprinted by permission.

Jesus' first miracle involved the transmutation of water into wine. Given the probable amount involved—120 gallons, according to Scripture scholars—after all the wine provided was already consumed, He not only began His public ministry, but scandalized generations of prigs from that time to this. He would repeat this feat (only ratcheting up the ante, turning wine to His own blood) at the Last Supper, instituting the central act of Christian worship and opening the door for centuries of controversy.

The Marriage Feast at Cana

And the third day, there was a marriage in Cana of Galilee: and the mother of Jesus was there.

And Jesus also was invited, and his disciples, to the marriage.

And the wine failing, the mother of Jesus saith to him: They have no wine.

And Jesus saith to her: Woman, what is that to me and to thee? My hour is not yet come. His mother saith to the waiters: Whatsover he shall say to you, do ye.

Now there were set six waterpots of stone, according to the manner of the Jews, containing two or three measures apiece.

Jesus saith to them: Fill the waterpots with water. And they filled them up to the brim.

And Jesus saith to them: Draw out now, and carry to the chief steward of the feast. And they carried it.

And when the chief steward had tasted the water made wine, and knew not whence it was, but the waiters knew who had drawn the water; the chief steward calleth the bridegroom,

And saith to him: Every man at first setteth forth good wine, and when men have drunk, then that which is worse. But thou has kept the good wine until now.

From *The Gospel of St. John*, chapter 2, verses 1–10, Douai-Rheims version.

4

Banquets such as the one described by Petronius were an enormous part of the Roman world's social life. The tenor of these entertainments may be gleaned from St. Clement of Alexandria's advice to Christians attending them. Do not vomit on your neighbor, *he ordered. He further commanded,* do not gulp all your wine at once. It has been given you, and will not be taken away. *Still good advice at public functions.*

Trimalchio's Banquet

Petronius Arbiter

Drunk with admiration, we brought up the rear and Agamemnon joined us when we reached Trimalchio's door. Beside the door we saw a sign:

ANY SLAVE LEAVING THE PREMISES
WITHOUT AUTHORIZATION FROM THE MASTER
WILL RECEIVE ONE HUNDRED LASHES!

At the entrance sat the porter, dressed in that same leek-green that seemed to be the livery of the house. A cherry-colored sash was bound around his waist and he was busily shelling peas into a pan of solid silver. In the doorway hung a cage, all gold, and in it a magpie was croaking out his welcome to the guests.

I was gaping at all this in open-mouthed wonder when I suddenly jumped with terror, stumbled, and nearly broke my leg. For there on the left as you entered, in fresco, stood a huge dog straining at his leash. In large letters under the painting was scrawled:

BEWARE OF THE DOG![1]

The others burst out laughing at my fright. But when I'd recovered from the shock, I found myself following the rest of the frescoes with fascination. They ran the whole length of the wall. First came a panel showing a slave market with everything

1. At Pompeii, in the entrance to the so-called House of the Tragic Poet, there is a splendid mosaic of a leashed dog and beneath it the inscription: CAVE CANEM ("BEWARE OF THE DOG").

clearly captioned. There stood Trimalchio as a young man, his hair long and curly in slave fashion; in his hand he held a staff[2] and he was entering Rome for the first time under the sponsorship of Minerva.[3] In the next panel he appeared as an apprentice accountant, then as a paymaster—each step in his career portrayed in great detail and everything scrupulously labeled. At the end of the portico you came to the climax of the series: a picture of Mercury grasping Trimalchio by the chin and hoisting him up to the lofty eminence of the official's tribunal.[4] Beside the dais stood the godess Fortuna with a great cornucopia and the three Fates, busily spinning out Trimalchio's life in threads of gold,[5] while in the background a group of runners were shown working out with their trainer. In the corner at the end of the portico was a huge wardrobe with a small built-in shrine. In the shrine were silver statuettes of the household gods, a Venus in marble, and a golden casket containing, I was told, the clippings from Trimalchio's first beard.[6] I began questioning the attendant about some other frescoes in the middle. "Scenes from the Iliad and the Odyssey," he explained, "and the gladiator games given by Laenas."[7] But there was far too little time to ask about everything that took my eye.

We approached the dining room next where we found the steward at the door making up his accounts. I was particularly struck by the doorposts. For fixed to the jamb were fasces,[8] bundles of sticks with axes protruding from them; but on the lower

2. The caduceus of Mercury, the god of trade and Trimalchio's special patron.

3. As goddess of crafts (and Wisdom?), Minerva conducts Trimalchio to Rome.

4. The seat to which Mercury hoists Trimalchio is the throne allotted to the Sevirs, that is, the officials appointed in the municipalities to carry out the worship of the deified Emperor. Election to this office was normally purchased, and Trimalchio was proud of having been appointed without payment.

5. They symbolize, of course, a life of gold.

6. The first trimming of the beard was regarded by Romans as symbolic of a boy's having attained his manhood and was usually the preliminary to his donning the man's garb, the toga virilis.

7. His gladiator games are otherwise unknown. Their presence here, however, is deliberately incongruous, an exposure of the vulgarity of taste of a man who could juxtapose scenes from Homer with others from mere gladiatorial games. The modern analogy would be the case of that book-collecting millionaire who claimed to specialize in "twelfth-century incunabula and first editions of Zane Grey."

8. In Republican times fasces were symbols of authority, borne by lictors (or bearers) in attendance upon a magistrate possessing the imperium. The rods signified the magistrate's power of administering a flogging; the ax, the power of life and death. Under the Empire, however, fasces were made available even to the Sevirs, each of whom was allowed two lictors.

side the bundles terminated in what looked like the brass ram of a ship,[9] and on the brass this inscription had been engraved:

TO GAIUS POMPEIUS TRIMALCHIO,
OFFICIAL OF THE IMPERIAL CULT,[10]
FROM HIS STEWARD
CINNAMUS.

Hanging from the ceiling on a long chain was a two-bracket lamp with the same inscription, and on each of the doorposts a wooden tablet had been put up. On one of these, if I remember rightly, this memo was written:

"The Master will be dining in town
on the 30th and 31st of December."[11]

On the other tablet was a diagram of the orbits of the moon and the seven planets, with the lucky and unlucky days all indicated by knobs of different colors.[12]

We duly noted these refinements and were just about to step into the dining room when suddenly a slave—clearly posted for this very job—shouted, "RIGHT FEET FIRST!" Well, needless to say, we froze. Who wants to bring down bad luck on his host by walking into his dining room in the wrong way?[13] However, we synchronized our legs and were just stepping out, right feet first, when a slave, utterly naked, landed on the floor in front of us and implored us to save him from a whipping. He

9. The meaning of these brass rams is uncertain. It may be merely that Trimalchio is again guilty of pretentious bad taste, or that he liked this imposing, semiofficial suggestion of naval triumph. As a man who had made enormous wealth from merchant-shipping, he could think of himself as having won some sort of naval triumph. And to get from that to the notion of himself as almost an admiral would not be beyond the limits of his ingenuity of pretensions. His only problem is to know how close he can sail to the letter of the law, without incurring its penalties.

10. That is, a Sevir.

11. The point of this memo would probably be clearer if we knew with certainty the date of Trimalchio's dinner. There are some hints that the date may be sometime in January. If so, the memo must be intended to show Trimalchio's social importance: he is so much in demand that he has to be booked for an invitation almost a year in advance of the date.

12. Superstition is one of Trimalchio's most prominent traits.

13. Romans regarded it as tempting fate to cross a threshold or begin a journey left foot first. Such a step, that is, was sinister (Latin for "left" and a bad presage). On the right, however, all was well.

was about to be flogged, he explained, for a trifling offense. He had let someone steal the steward's clothing, worthless stuff really, in the baths. Well, we pulled back our right feet, faced about and returned to the entry where we found the steward counting a stack of gold coins. We begged him to let the servant off. "Really, it's not the money I mind," he replied with enormous condescension, "so much as the idiot's carelessness. It was my dinner-suit he lost, a birthday present from one of my dependents. Expensive too, but then I've already had it washed. Well, it's a trifle.[14] Do what you want with him." We thanked him for his gracious kindness, but when we entered the dining room up ran the same slave whom we'd just begged off. He overwhelmed us with his thanks and then, to our consternation, began to plaster us with kisses. "You'll soon see whom you've helped," he said. "The master's wine will prove the servant's gratitude."

At last we took our places. Immediately slaves from Alexandria came in and poured ice water[15] over our hands. These were followed by other slaves who knelt at our feet and with extraordinary skill pedicured our toenails. Not for an instant, moreover, during the whole of this odious job, did one of them stop singing. This made me wonder whether the whole menage was given to bursts of song, so I put it to the test by calling for a drink. It was served immediately by a boy who trilled away as shrilly as the rest of them. In fact, anything you asked for was invariably served with a snatch of song, so that you would have thought you were eating in a concert-hall rather than a private dining room.

Now that the guests were all in their places, the hors d'oeuvres were served, and very sumptuous they were. Trimalchio alone was still absent, and the place of honor—reserved for the host in modern fashion—stood empty.[16] But I was speaking

14. Expensive because dyed with the famous Tyrian dye. This dye (its color is commonly supposed to have been "royal purple," but judging from modern experiments it comes closer to a rich-reddish brown, the color of dried blood) was fabulously expensive and only the very richest could afford it. Petronius' point is that Trimalchio's wealth is on such an astronomical scale that not only does he have a steward who has dependents (clientes) so rich that they can present him with clothing worth a king's ransom, but that the steward himself is so fabulously rich that he can, as a favor to his master's guests, forgive the loss of his clothing as a mere trifle.

15. Three seasons out of the year, especially in Roman times, ice water would be a great luxury. During the Italian winter, however, it is supplied in bitter abundance.

16. It is difficult to explain the probable seating arrangements in effect at this particular dinner. The conventional arrangement calls for nine diners (or fewer), but if we assume that two diners shared the same couch or that there were other tables, the difficulty disappears. At dinner each guest was assigned a couch,

of the hors d'oeuvres. On a large tray stood a donkey made of rare Corinthian bronze[17]; on the donkey's back were two panniers, one holding green olives, the other, black. Flanking the donkey were two side dishes, both engraved with Trimalchio's name and the weight of the silver, while in dishes shaped to resemble little bridges there were dormice,[18] all dipped in honey and rolled in poppyseed. Nearby, on a silver grill, piping hot, lay small sausages, while beneath the grill black damsons and red pomegranates had been sliced up and arranged so as to give the effect of flames playing over charcoal.

We were nibbling at these splendid appetizers when suddenly the trumpets blared a fanfare and Trimalchio was carried in,[19] propped up on piles of miniature pillows in such a comic way that some of us couldn't resist impolitely smiling. His head, cropped close in a recognizable slave cut, protruded from a cloak of blazing scarlet; his neck, heavily swathed already in bundles of clothing was wrapped in a large napkin bounded by an incongruous senatorial purple stripe with little tassels dangling down here and there. On the little finger of his left hand he sported an immense gilt ring; the ring on the last joint of his fourth finger looked to be solid gold of the kind the lesser nobility wear, but was actually, I think, an imitation, pricked out with small steel stars. Nor does this exhaust the inventory of his trinkets. At least he

---

and the couches themselves were grouped by threes around the three sides of a large table. Dinner was eaten from a reclining position; the diner supported his head with his left arm, elbow on the table, and ate with his right hand. The free side of the table was used for serving and carving, and the table itself must have been lower than the couches where the diners ate.

17. A famous bronze alloy, very highly prized by ancient connoisseurs—including Trimalchio. Its composition is unknown.

18. Small rodents intermediate between the mouse and the squirrel; they were regarded as a great delicacy in antiquity.

19. Trimalchio's entrance deserves comment. It is primarily the elaborate incongruity of his dress that accounts for the amusement of the more sophisticated guests. Thus, while the close-cropped haircut is typical of the slave or the recently manumitted slave, the broad purple stripe was a privilege permitted only to the Senatorial class. The gold rings, on the other hand, are the prerogative of the equestrian order. Trimalchio, having the right to neither the broad purple stripe nor the equestrian ring, does the next best thing, wearing an imitation steel ring and transferring the purple stripe from the toga to the napkin. Presumably, those who adopted insignia to which they had no legal right could be punished. For this reason Trimalchio specifies that the statue of himself on his tomb is to be shown wearing "five gold rings": the fraud would be unpunishable after death. The tassels may be a sign of effeminacy. The silver toothpick, of course, is sheer extravagance.

rather ostentatiously bared his arm to show us a large gold bracelet and ivory circlet with a shiny metal plate.

He was picking his teeth with a silver toothpick when he first addressed us. "My friends," he said, "I wasn't anxious to eat just yet, but I've ignored my own wishes so as not to keep you waiting. Still, perhaps you won't mind if I finish my game." At these words a slave jumped forward with a board of juniper wood and a pair of crystal dice. I noticed one other elegant novelty as well: in place of the usual black and white counters, Trimalchio had substituted gold and silver coins. His playing, I might add, was punctuated throughout with all sorts of vulgar exclamations.

We, meanwhile, were still occupied with the hors d'oeuvres when a tray was carried in and set down before us. On it lay a basket, and in it a hen, carved from wood, with wings outspread as though sitting on her eggs. Then two slaves came forward and, to a loud flourish from the orchestra, began rummaging in the straw and pulling out peahen's eggs[20] which they divided among the guests. Trimalchio gave the whole performance his closest attention. "Friends," he said, "I ordered peahen eggs to be set under that hen, but I'm half afraid they may have hatched already. Still, let's see if we can suck them." We were handed spoons—weighing at least half a pound apiece—and cracked open the eggs, which turned out to be baked from rich pastry. To tell the truth, I had almost tossed my share away, thinking the eggs were really addled. But I heard one of the guests, obviously a veteran of these dinners, say, "I wonder what little surprise we've got in here." So I cracked the shell with my hand and found inside a fine fat oriole,[21] nicely seasoned with pepper.

By this time Trimalchio had finished his game. He promptly sent for the same dishes we had had and with a great roaring voice offered a second cup of mead to anyone who wanted it. Then the orchestra suddenly blared and the trays were snatched away from the tables by a troupe of warbling waiters. But in the confusion a silver side dish fell to the floor. Immediately the servant in charge of the dishware came pattering up with a broom and swept the silver dish out the door with the rest of the rubbish. Two curly-haired Ethiopian slaves followed him as he swept, both car-

---

20. A fabulous delicacy.

21. Actually, the Latin gives ficedula, the modern Italian beccafico or fig-eater, a brilliantly colored bird whose habit of stuffing itself on ripe figs endeared it to Roman epicures. Since the fig-eater is unknown in America, I have translated it "oriole," to which family it belongs.

rying little skin bottles like the circus attendants who sprinkle the arena with perfume, and poured wine over our hands. No one was offered water.

We clapped enthusiastically for this fine display of extravagance. "The god of war," said Trimalchio, "is a real democrat.[22] That's why I gave orders that each of us should have a table to himself. Besides, these stinking slaves will bother us less than if we were all packed in together."

Glass jars carefully sealed and coated were now brought in. Each bore this label:

GENUINE FALERNIAN WINE
GUARANTEED ONE HUNDRED YEARS
OLD!
BOTTLED
IN THE CONSULSHIP
OF
OPIMIUS.[23]

While we were reading the labels, Trimalchio clapped his hands for attention. "Just think, friends, wine lasts longer than us poor suffering humans. So soak it up, it's the stuff of life. I give you, gentlemen, the genuine Opimian vintage. Yesterday I served much cheaper stuff and the guests were much more important." While we were commenting on it and savoring the luxury, a slave brought in a skeleton,[24] cast of solid silver, and fastened in such a way that the joints could be twisted and bent in any direction. The servants threw it down on the table in front of us and pushed it

---

22. The proverb means simply that in war (where all men face death alike), social distinctions vanish. Trimalchio, as usual, misapplies his proverbs.

23. Trimalchio's attempts to impress his guests commonly founder on ignorance. Here either his chronology or his knowledge of wines is at fault; probably both. Opimius was consul in 121 B.C., and assuming the date of the dinner is sometime during the reign of Nero, the wine—if Opimian—could not be much less than 170 years old. Opimian, in any case, was not a wine that kept well; like any other good Falernian, it began to deteriorate after twenty years.

24. The memento mori was a common part of Roman feasts or even of the decoration of the dining room. We still possess, for instance, a number of vivid mosaics portraying skeletons with eating vessels or food and a moralizing inscription. The point of these mementos, of course, was: "Eat, drink and be merry, for tomorrow we die." Trimalchio's memento is, one suspects, rather more vivid than usual, and the silver joints of the skeleton show the master's touch.

into several suggestive postures by twisting its joints, while Trimalchio recited this verse of his own making:

> Nothing but bones, that's what we are.
> Death hustles us humans away.
> Today we're here and tomorrow we're not,
> so live and drink while you may!

The course that followed our applause failed, however, to measure up to our expectations of our host, but it was so unusual that it took everybody's attention. Spaced around a circular tray were the twelve signs of the zodiac, and over each sign the chef had put the most appropriate food. [25] Thus, over the sign of Aries were chickpeas, over Taurus a slice of beef, a pair of testicles and kidneys over Gemini, a wreath of flowers over Cancer, over Leo an African fig, virgin sowbelly on Virgo, over Libra a pair of scales with a tartlet in one pan and a cheesecake in the other, over Scorpion a crawfish, a lobster on Capricorn, on Aquarius a goose, and two mullets over the sign of the Fishes. The centerpiece was a clod of turf with the grass still green on top and the whole thing surmounted by a fat honeycomb. Meanwhile, bread in a silver chafing dish was being handed around by a black slave with long hair who was shrilling in an atrocious voice some song from the pantomime called Asafoetida. With some reluctance we began to attack this wretched fare, but Trimalchio kept urging us, "Eat up, gentlemen, eat up!"

 A place where everybody from ballet dancers to iron workers to Wall Street brokers feels comfortable elbow to elbow.
—GERARD MEAGHER, OLD TOWN BAR, 45 E. 18TH STREET, NEW YORK

"Dinner With Trimalchio," from *The Satyricon* by Petronius, translated by William Arrowsmith, copyright © 1959, renewed © 1987 by William Arrowsmith. Used by permission of Dutton Signet, a division of Penguin Putnam, Inc.

25. In almost all cases, the link between the zodiacal sign and the food placed upon it is a pun or some farfetched resemblance. Thus beef is appropriate to Taurus (the Bull); thus over the Ram (Aries), one finds chickpeas (*cicer arietinus*), and so forth.

The Seven Sages of the Bamboo Grove were a group of Chinese scholars and poets of the mid-third century A.D.who banded together to escape from the hypocrisy and danger of the official world to a life of drinking wine and writing verse in the country. There they spent their days on the estate of a comrade of theirs, Hsi Kang, who had been wrongfully executed by the petty ruler of the state of Wei. Whiling away the time in drinking, talking, and writing poetry, they contemplated nature and the generally unpleasant nature of human affairs. In addition to Ruan, the company also featured one Liu Ling, whom the Brittanica *describes as "the confirmed drunkard." One can only guess what this title might have meant in that context!*

Xiuxi Yin

Ruan Ji

Fleeting worldly affairs have a ridiculous urgency;
   quiet and sad feelings are wasted heartache.
How does one resolve sadness? The answer is wine;
   being drunk all day allows a disregard for social etiquette.
During the 36,000 days of a century;
   one should drink 300 goblets of wine each day.
Such pleasure, to enter the Land of Drunkenness,
   First sober, then drunk; drunken and wild.
Once we have gone into the hills, we can immediately forget about worldly affairs.

In the sky there is a wine star, on earth a wine spring;
   from my walking stick I often hang a bag of coins.
A pool of wine with a mound of wine sediment alongside brings me pleasure,
   so I whirl about and drunkenly dance;
it is as if I am donning the feather cape,

donning the feather cape and ascending into immortality.
While in the cups I attain the Way in a truly joyful manner.

For wine I'd not regret swapping a valuable fur coat;
   when drinking with friends I can shed long-standing depression.
The dregs of fine wine in grand cups allow me to loosen my robe and relax;
   a great song brings lasting pleasure.
For worldly pleasure, nothing is better than wine.
   The pleasure of wine has a truly special quality.
In fact, after becoming drunk you can look askance at official duties.

As strong wine cooks the plump purple crabs,
   friends are called together to swig from their cups.
Whether taking pleasure in the mountains or streams,
   we don't concern ourselves with worldly affairs;
or even more, whether there is order or chaos,
   order or chaos and peace or danger.
A drunken man will fall down by himself; he doesn't need a push.

Once drunk, a cup of wine can bring 100 stanzas of poetry;
   and prized calligraphy strokes fill the paper.
In the Chang An market, (Li Bai) slept in a wine house.
   When the emperor summoned him and sent a boat to pick him up, Li Bai
     didn't get on it.
He said of himself, this humble servant is an immortal in his wine.

The old mountain man vomits his wine with the sound, "kuan, kuan";
   achieving fame and wealth is of no interest to him.
Liu Li, Bi Zhuo and Tao Qian all had correct manners and a lofty attitude.
   These people did not submit to government control;
(instead) they remained together in humble circumstances, relying on each
     other.

While the rest of society is drunk, I remain sober.
   (unlike others) I use wine to distance myself from disasters.
Of course I am not really addicted to drinking,

or being dissolute, becoming (like a common) drunken person.
Of old many illustrious people all remained unknown,
    it is only the drinkers who have left their name.
(This is because) an old toper's aim does not have to do with wine
    (but with achieving an elevated condition).

Translated from the Chinese by John Thompson, and accessible on his Web site at http://www.iohk.com/
UserPages/thompson/04sqmp/sq10jk.htm#f8

Xiuxi Yin

Although separated from us by a millennium, the Vikings of this tale were beset by many of the same ills affecting party-givers and -goers today. Not least of these, of course, is vomiting, which, however, in true Viking fashion is coupled with sword-play.

Egil's Saga

King Eirik and Gunnhild arrived in Atloy the same night. Bard had prepared a feast for him, because a sacrifice was being made to the disir. It was a splendid feast, with plenty to drink in the main room.

The king asked where Bard was.

'I can't see him anywhere,' he said.

'Bard is outside,' someone told him, 'serving his guests.'

'Who are these guests that he feels more obliged to attend to than to be in here with us?' asked the king.

The man told him that Thorir the Hersir's men were there.

'Go to them immediately and call them in here,' the king said.

This was done, and they were told the king wanted to meet them.

When they entered, the king welcomed Olvir, offering him a place at table opposite him in the high seat, with his men further down. They took their seats, and Egil sat next to Olvir.

Then the ale was served. Many toasts were drunk, each involving a whole ale-horn. As the night wore on, many of Olvir's companions became incapacitated; some of them vomited inside the main room, while others made it through the door. Bard insisted on serving them more drink.

Egil took the drinking-horn that Bard had given to Olvir and finished it off. Saying that Egil was clearly very thirsty, Bard gave him another full horn at once and asked him to drink that too. Egil took the horn and spoke a verse:

> 8. You told the trollwomen's foe[1]
>   you were short of feast-drink

1. trollwomen's foe: noble man.

when appeasing the goddesses:
You deceived us, despoiler of graves.
You hid your plotting thoughts
from men you did not know
for sheer spite, Bard:
you have played a bad trick on us.

Bard told Egil to stop mocking him and get on with his drinking. Egil drank every draught that was handed to him, and those meant for Olvir too.

Then Bard went up to the queen and told her that this man was bringing shame on them, always claiming to be thirsty no matter how much he drank. The queen and Bard mixed poison into the drink and brought it in. Bard made a sign over the draught and handed it to the serving woman, who took it to Egil and offered him a drink. Egil took out his knife and stabbed the palm of his hand with it, then took the drinking-horn, carved runes on it and smeared them with blood. He spoke a verse:

9. I carve runes on this horn,
   redden words with my blood,
   I choose words for the trees[2]
   of the wild beast's ear-roots[3];
   drink as we wish this mead
   brought by merry servants,
   let us find out how we fare
   from the ale that Bard blessed.

The horn shattered and the drink spilled on to the straw. Olvir was on the verge of passing out, so Egil got up and led him over to the door. He swung his cloak over his shoulder and gripped his sword underneath it. When they reached the door, Bard went after them with a full horn and asked Olvir to drink a farewell toast. Egil stood in the doorway and spoke this verse:

10. I'm feeling drunk, and the ale
    has left Olvir pale in the gills,
    I let the spray of ox-spears[4]

2. their trees: horns.
3. ear-roots: part of the head.
4. ox-spears: drinking-horns.

foam over my beard.
Your wits have gone, inviter
of showers on to shield;
now the rain[5] of the high god
starts pouring upon you.

Egil tossed away the horn, grabbed hold of his sword and drew it. It was dark in the doorway; he thrust the sword so deep into Bard's stomach that the point came out through his back. Bard fell down dead, blood pouring from the wound. Then Olvir dropped to the floor, spewing vomit. Egil ran out of the room. It was pitch-dark outside, and he dashed from the farm.

People left the room and saw Bard and Olvir lying on the floor together, and imagined at first that they had killed each other. Because it was dark, the king had a light brought over, and they could see that Olvir was lying unconscious in his vomit, but Bard had been killed, and the floor was awash with his blood.

The king asked where that huge man was who had drunk the most that night, and was told that he had gone out in front of Olvir.

'Search for him,' ordered the king, 'and bring him to me.'

A search was made for him around the farm, but he was nowhere to be found. When the king's men went into the fire-room where they had been eating that night, many of Olvir's men were lying there on the floor and others up against the wall of the house. They asked whether Egil had been there. They were told he had run in and taken his weapons, then gone back out.

Then they went into the main room and reported this to the king, who ordered his men to act quickly and take all the ships that were on the island, 'and tomorrow when it is light we will comb the whole island and kill that man.'

 Between the laid-back atmosphere, top-notch cocktails, and eclectic all-American wine list, the Grange Hall is a great place to meet for a drink.
—DOUG MARKS, BARTENDER, THE GRANGE HALL, 50 COMMERCE STREET, NEW YORK

From *The Sagas of Icelanders*, 2000. Reykjavik: Leifur Eiriksson Publishing, pp. 67–69.

5. rain: i.e., of spears, perhaps of poetry (or vomit?).

Seven centuries passed from the time of the Vikings to their eighteenth-century English partial descendants. But as the following chapter from Tom Jones *makes clear, the passage of time did little either to quench their thirst or to sharpen their wits. Then again, poor Tom might have had trouble in any age, powdered wig or not.*

Tom Jones, Chapter IX

Henry Fielding

Which, among other Things, may serve as a Comment on that Saying of Aeschines, that DRUNKENNESS SHEWS THE MIND OF A MAN, AS A MIRROUR RE-FLECTS HIS PERSON

The reader may, perhaps, wonder at hearing nothing of Mr. Jones in the last chapter. In fact, his behavior was so different from that of the persons there mentioned, that we chose not to confound his name with theirs.

When the good man had ended his speech, Jones was the last who deserted the room. Thence he retired to his own apartment, to give vent to his concern; but the restlessness of his mind would not suffer him to remain long there; he slipped softly, therefore, to Allworthy's chamber door, where he listened a considerable time without hearing any kind of motion within, unless a violent snoring, which at last his fears misrepresented as groans. This so alarmed him, that he could not forbear entering the room; where he found the good man in the bed, in a sweet composed sleep, and his nurse snoring in the above-mentioned hearty manner, at the bed's feet. He immediately took the only method of silencing this thorough bass, whose music he feared might disturb Mr. Allworthy; and then sitting down by the nurse, he remained motionless till Blifil and the doctor came in together, and waked the sick man; in order that the doctor might feel his pulse, and that the other might communicate to him that piece of news, which, had Jones been apprised of it, would have had great difficulty of finding its way to Mr. Allworthy's ear at such a season.

When he first heard Blifil tell his uncle this story, Jones could hardly contain the wrath which kindled in him at the other's indiscretion, especially as the doctor shook his head, and declared his unwillingness to have the matter mentioned to his patient. But as his passion did not so far deprive him of all use of his understanding, as to hide from him the consequences which any violent expressions towards Blifil might have on the sick, this apprehension stilled his rage, at the present; and he grew afterwards so satisfied with finding that his news had, in fact, produced no mischief, that he suffered his anger to die in his own bosom, without ever mentioning it to Blifil.

The physician dined that day at Mr Allworthy's; and having after dinner visited his patient, he returned to the company, and told them, that he had now the satisfaction to say, with assurance, that his patient was out of all danger: that he had brought his fever to a perfect intermission, and doubted not by throwing in the bark to prevent its return.

This account so pleased Jones, and threw him into such immoderate excess of rapture, that he might be truly said to be drunk with joy. An intoxication which greatly forwards the effects of wine; and as he was very free too with the bottle on this occasion, (for he drank many bumpers to the doctor's health, as well as to other toasts) he became very soon literally drunk.

Jones had naturally violent animal spirits: these being set on float, and augmented by the spirit of wine, produced most extravagant effects. He kissed the doctor, and embraced him with the most passionate endearments; swearing that, next to Mr. Allworthy himself, he loved him of all men living. 'Doctor,' added he, 'you deserve a statue to be erected to you at the public expense, for having preserved a man, who is not only the darling of all good men who know him, but a blessing to society, the glory of his country, and an honor to human nature. D—n me if I don't love him better than my own soul.'

'More shame for you,' cries Thwackum. 'Though I think you have reason to love him, for he hath provided very well for you. And, perhaps, it might have been better for some folks, that he had not lived to see just reason of revoking his gift.'

Jones now, looking on Thwackum with inconceivable disdain, answered, 'And doth thy mean soul imagine, that any such considerations could weigh with me? No, let the earth open and swallow her own dirt (if I had millions of acres I would say it) rather than swallow up my dear glorious friend.'

Quis desiderio sit pudor aut modus
Tam chari capitis?

The doctor now interposed, and prevented the effects of a wrath which was kindling between Jones and Thwackum; after which the former gave a loose to mirth, sang two or three amorous songs, and fell into every frantic disorder which unbridled joy is apt to inspire; but so far was he from any disposition to quarrel, that he was ten times better humored, if possible, than when he was sober.

To say truth, nothing is more erroneous than the common observation, that men who are ill-natured and quarrelsome when they are drunk, are very worthy persons when they are sober: for drink, in reality, doth not reverse nature, or create passions in men which did not exist in them before. It takes away the guard of reason, and consequently forces us to produce those symptoms which many, when sober, have art enough to conceal. It heightens and inflames our passions, (generally indeed that passion which is uppermost in our mind) so that the angry temper, the amorous, the generous, the good-humored, the avaricious, and all other dispositions of men, are in their cups heightened and exposed.

And yet no nation produces so many drunken quarrels, especially among the lower people, as England; (for, indeed, with them, to drink and to fight together, are almost synonymous terms) I would not, methinks, have it thence concluded, that the English are the worst-natured people alive. Perhaps the love of glory only is at the bottom of this; so that the fair conclusion seems to be, that our countrymen have more of that love, and more of bravery, than any other plebeians. And this the rather, as there is seldom anything ungenerous, unfair, or ill-natured, exercised on those occasions: nay, it is common for the combatants to express good-will for each other, even at the time of the conflict; and as their drunken mirth generally ends in a battle, so do most of their battles end in friendship.

But to return to our history. Though Jones had shown no design of giving offense, yet Mr. Blifil was highly offended at a behavior which was so inconsistent with the sober and prudent reserve of his own temper. He bore it too with the greater impatience, as it appeared to him very indecent at this season; 'When,' as he said, 'the house was a house of mourning, on the account of his dear mother; and if it had pleased Heaven to give them some prospect of Mr. Allworthy's recovery, it would become them better to express the exultations of their hearts in thanksgiving, than in drunkenness and riots; which were properer methods to increase the Divine wrath, than to avert it.' Thwackum, who had swallowed more liquor than Jones, but without any ill effect on his brain, seconded the pious harangue of Blifil: but Square, for reasons which the reader may probably guess, was totally silent.

Wine had not so totally overpowered Jones, as to prevent his recollecting Mr. Blifil's loss, the moment it was mentioned. As no person, therefore, was more ready to confess and condemn his own errors, he offered to shake Mr. Blifil by the hand, and begged his pardon, saying 'His excessive joy for Mr. Allworthy's recovery had driven every other thought out of his mind.'

Blifil scornfully rejected his hand; and, with much indignation, answered, 'It was little to be wondered at, if tragical spectacles made no impression on the blind; but, for his part, he had the misfortune to know who his parents were, and consequently must be affected with their loss.'

Jones, who, notwithstanding his good humor, had some mixture of the irascible in his constitution, leaped hastily from his chair, and catching hold of Blifil's collar, cried out, 'D—n you for a rascal, do you insult me with the misfortune of my birth?' He accompanied these words with such rough actions, that they soon got the better of Mr. Blifil's peaceful temper; and a scuffle immediately ensued, which might have produced mischief, had it not been prevented by the interposition of Thwackum and the physician; for the philosophy of Square rendered him superior to all emotions, and he very calmly smoked his pipe, as was his custom in all broils, unless when he apprehended some danger of having it broke in his mouth.

The combatants being now prevented from executing present vengeance on each other, betook themselves to the common resources of disappointed rage, and vented their wrath in threats and defiance. In this kind of conflict, Fortune, which in the personal attack, seemed to incline to Jones, was now altogether as favorable to his enemy.

A truce, nevertheless, was at length agreed on, by the mediation of the neutral parties, and the whole company again sat down at the table; where Jones being prevailed on to ask pardon, and Blifil to give it, peace was restored, and everything seemed in statu quo.

But though the quarrel was, in all appearance, perfectly reconciled, the good-humor which had been interrupted by it, was by no means restored. All merriment was now at an end, and the subsequent discourse consisted only of grave relations of matters of fact, and of as grave observations upon them. A species of conversation, in which, though there is much of dignity and instruction, there is but little entertainment. As we presume, therefore, only to convey this last to the reader, we shall pass by whatever was said, till the rest of the company having, by degrees, dropped off, left

Square and the physician only together; at which time the conversation was a little heightened by some comments on what had happened between the two young gentlemen; both of whom the doctor declared to be no better than scoundrels; to which appellation the philosopher, very sagaciously shaking his head, agreed.

Tom Jones, originally published in 1749, Bantam Classic Edition published in July 1997, pp. 253–258.

The French are a wise race; your editor hopes he does not think so solely because he himself is of French descent. Nevertheless, this excerpt from Brillat-Savarin's Physiology of Taste *shows the dry wit and good sense for which both he and his nationality are renowned.*

On Drinks

Jean-Anthelme Brillat-Savarin

52. INTRODUCTION

The word drink is used of any liquid which can be used to accompany our food.

Water seems to be the most natural drink. It is found wherever there are animals, takes the place of milk among adults, and is no less necessary to us than air.

WATER

Water is the only drink which really quenches thirst, and that is the reason why it can only be drunk in comparatively small quantities. Most of the other liquors which man imbibes are only palliatives, and if he had confined himself to water, it would never have been said of him that one of his privileges was to drink without being thirsty.

THE PROMPT EFFECT OF DRINKS

Drinks are absorbed into the animal economy with extreme ease; their effect is prompt, and the relief which they give almost instantaneous. Lay a substantial meal before a tired man, and he will eat with difficulty and be little the better for it at first. Give him a glass of wine or brandy, and immediately he feels better: you see him come to life again before you.

A curious occurrence, of which my nephew, Colonel Guigard, told me, lends support to this theory. My nephew is no storyteller by nature, but the truth of his tale is beyond question.

He was at the head of a detachment returning from the siege of Jaffa, and they had reached a point only a few hundred paces from the place where they were due to make a halt and find some water when they noticed some dead bodies on the road; they were the corpses of some soldiers belonging to a detachment a day's march ahead of my nephew's, who had died of the heat.

Among the victims of that burning climate was a carabineer who was known to several of my nephew's men. He had presumably been dead for over twenty-four hours, and the sun, beating down on him all day, had turned his face as black as a crow.

Some of his comrades came over to the body, either to look at him one last time, or to collect their inheritance, if there was anything to inherit; and they were astonished to find his limbs still flexible; and even a little warmth in the neighborhood of the heart.

'Give him a drop of *sacre-chien*,' said the wag of the detachment; 'I'll bet that unless he's gone a long way into the next world, he'll come back for a taste of that.'

Sure enough, at the first spoonful of spirits the dead man opened his eyes; everyone cried out in amazement; and after his temples had been rubbed with the spirits and he had been given a little more to drink, he was able, with some assistance, to keep his seat on a donkey.

They led him like this to the well; during the night he was looked after carefully, and given a few dates to eat, with some other light food; and the following day, again mounted on the donkey, he reached Cairo with the rest.

53. STRONG DRINKS

A thing of enormous interest is that sort of instinct, as general as it is imperious, which leads us in search of strong drinks.

Wine, the most delightful of drinks, whether we owe it to Noah, who planted the vine, or to Bacchus, who pressed juice from the grape, dates from the childhood of the world; and beer, which is attributed to Osiris, goes back to a period beyond which nothing certain is known.

All men, even those it is customary to call savages, have been so tormented by this craving for strong drinks, that they have always managed to obtain them, however limited the extent of their knowledge.

They have turned the milk of their domestic animals sour, or extracted juice from various fruits and roots which they suspected of containing the elements of fermentation; and wherever human society has existed, we find that men were provided with strong liquors, which they used at their feasts, sacrifices, marriages, or funerals, in short on all occasions of merry-making or solemnity.

Wine was drunk and its praises sung for many centuries before men guessed at the possibility of extracting the spirituous part which makes its strength; but when the Arabs taught us the art of distillation, which they had invented for the purpose of extracting the scent of flowers, and above all that of the rose which occupies such an important place in their writings, then men began to believe that it was possible to discover in wine the cause of that special savor which has such a stimulating influence on the organ of taste; and so, step by step, alcohol, spirits of wine, and brandy were discovered.

Alcohol is the prince of liquids, and carries the palate to its highest pitch of exaltation; its various preparations have opened up a new source of pleasure; it invests certain medicaments with a power which they could not otherwise have attained; and it has even become a formidable weapon in our hands, for the nations of the New World have been subdued and destroyed almost as much by brandy as by firearms.

The method by which alcohol was discovered has led to other important results; for consisting as it does in the separation and exposure of the parts which make up a body, and distinguish that body from all others, it has served as a model to scholars pursuing analogous researches; and they have made known to us entirely new substances, such as strychnine, quinine, morphine, and others, both discovered and to be discovered in the future.

Be that as it may, this thirst for a kind of liquid which Nature has enveloped in veils, this strange desire that assails all the races of mankind, in every climate and temperature, is most worthy to attract the attention of the philosophic observer.

I, among others, have pondered it, and I am tempted to place the craving for fermented liquors, which is unknown to animals, with anxiety regarding the future, which is likewise unknown to animals, and to regard both as distinctive attributes of the masterpiece of the last sublunary revolution.

If you are feeling happy or sad; if it's day or night, you can always come to the Smoke House, where the mood is always right.

—Israel "Izzy" Aviles, floor manager, Smoke House Restaurant, 4420 Lakeside Drive, Burbank, California

From *The Philosopher in the Kitchen,* Jean-Anthelme Brillat-Savarin, translated by Anne Drayton. Originally published in 1825; this edition, 1970. New York: Penguin Books, pp. 126–129. Published by Penguin Books in 1970, pp. 126–129.

Never was there so convivial a time as Christmas, nor so genial a writer as our own Washington Irving. Here we see a Yuletide banquet as we wish it would be: lubricated and jolly, and never descending into bickering and vomit! This is as far a cry from the Hallowe'en antics of the Headless Horseman as one could imagine.

The Christmas Dinner

Washington Irving

Lo, now is come our joyful'st feast!
Let every man be jolly,
Eache roome with yvie leaves is drest,
And every post with holly.
Now all our neighbours' chimneys smoke,
And Christmas blocks are burning;
Their ovens they with bak't meats choke,
And all their spits are turning.
Without the door let sorrow lie,
An if, for cold, it hap to die,
Wee 'l bury 't in a Christmas pye,
And evermore be merry.

Wither's Juvenilia

I had finished my toilet, and was loitering with Frank Bracebridge in the library, when we heard a distant thwacking sound, which he informed me was a signal for the serving up of the dinner. The Squire kept up old customs in kitchen as well as hall; and the rolling-pin struck upon the dresser by the cook, summoned the servants to carry in the meats.

Just in the nick the cook knock'd thrice,
And all the waiters in a trice

His summons did obey;
Each serving man, with dish in hand,
March'd boldly up, like our train band,
Presented, and away. (Sir John Suckling)

The dinner was served up in the great hall, where the Squire always held his Christmas banquet. A blazing, crackling fire of logs had been heaped on to warm the spacious apartment, and the flame went sparkling and wreathing up the wide-mouthed chimney. The great picture of the crusader and his white horse had been profusely decorated with greens for the occasion; and holly and ivy had likewise been wreathed round the helmet and weapons on the opposite wall, which I understood were the arms of the same warrior. I must own, by the by, I had strong doubts about the authenticity of the painting and armor as having belonged to the crusader, they certainly having the stamp of more recent days; but I was told that the painting had been so considered time out of mind; and that, as to the armor, it had been found in a lumber-room, and elevated to its present situation by the Squire, who at once de-termined it to be the armor of the family hero; and as he was absolute authority on all such subjects in his own household, the matter had passed into current acceptation. A sideboard was set out just under this chivalric trophy, on which was a display of plate that might have vied (at least in variety) with Belshazzar's parade of the vessels of the temple: "flagons, cans, cups, beakers, goblets, basins, and ewers"; the gorgeous utensils of good companionship that had gradually accumulated through many gen-erations of jovial housekeepers. Before these stood the two Yule candles, beaming like two stars of the first magnitude; other lights were distributed in branches, and the whole array glittered like a firmament of silver.

We were ushered into this banqueting scene with the sound of minstrelsy, the old harper being seated on a stool beside the fireplace, and twanging his instrument with a vast deal more power than melody. Never did Christmas board display a more goodly and gracious assemblage of countenances; those who were not handsome were, at least, happy; and happiness is a rare improver of your hard-favored visage. I always consider an old English family as well worth studying as a collection of Holbein's portraits or Albert Durer's prints. There is much antiquarian lore to be ac-quired; much knowledge of the physiognomies of former times. Perhaps it may be from having continually before their eyes those rows of old family portraits, with which the mansions of this country are stocked; certain it is, that the quaint features of antiquity are often most faithfully perpetuated in these ancient lines; and I have traced an old family nose through a whole picture gallery, legitimately handed down from generation to generation, almost from the time of the Conquest. Something of the kind was to be observed in the worthy company around me. Many of their faces had evidently originated in a Gothic age, and been merely copied by succeeding generations; and there was one little girl in particular, of staid demeanor, with a high Roman nose, and an antique vinegar aspect, who was a great favorite of the Squire's being, as he said, a Bracebridge all over, and the very counterpart of one of his ancestors who figured in the court of Henry VIII.

The parson said grace, which was not a short familiar one, such as is commonly addressed to the Deity in these unceremonious days; but a long, courtly, well-worded one of the ancient school. There was now a pause, as if something was expected; when suddenly the butler entered the hall with some degree of bustle: he was attended by a servant on each side with a large wax-light, and bore a silver dish, on which was an enormous pig's head, decorated with rosemary, with a lemon it its mouth, which was placed with great formality at the head of the table. The moment this pageant made its appearance, the harper struck up a flourish; at the conclusion of which the young Oxonian, on receiving a hint from the Squire, gave, with an air of the most comic gravity, an old carol, the first verse of which was as follows:—

> Caput apri defero
> Reddens laudes Domino.
> The boar's head in hand bring I,
> With garlands gay and rosemary.
> I pray you all synge merrily
> Qui estis in convivio.

Though prepared to witness many of these little eccentricities, from being apprised of the peculiar hobby of mine host, yet, I confess, the parade with which so odd a dish was introduced somewhat perplexed me, until I gathered from the conversation of the Squire and the parson, that it was meant to represent the bringing in of the boar's head: a dish formerly served up with much ceremony and the sound of minstrelsy and song, at great tables, on Christmas day. "I like the old custom," said the Squire, "not merely because it is stately and pleasing in itself, but because it was observed at the college at Oxford at which I was educated. When I hear the old song chanted, it brings to mind the time when I was young and gamesome,—and the noble old college-hall,—and my fellow-students loitering about in their black gowns; many of whom, poor lads, are now in their graves!"

The parson, however, whose mind was not haunted by such associations, and who was always more taken up with the text than the sentiment, objected to the Oxonian's version of the carol; which he affirmed was different from that sung at college. He went on, with the dry perseverance of a commentator, to give the college reading, accompanied by sundry annotations; addressing himself at first to the company at large; but finding their attention gradually diverted to other talk and other objects, he lowered his tone as his number of auditors diminished, until he concluded his remarks in an undervoice, to a fatheaded old gentleman next to him, who was silently engaged in the discussion of a huge plateful of turkey. (Footnote: The old ceremony of serving up the boar's head on Christmas day is still observed in the hall of Queen's College, Oxford. I was favored by the parson with a copy of the carol as now sung, and, as it may be acceptable to such of my readers as are curious in these grave and learned matters, I give it entire.)

The boar's head in hand bear I,
Bedeck'd with bays and rosemary;
And I pray you, my masters, be merry
Quot estis in convivio.
Caput apri defero,
Reddens laudes domino.

The boar's head, as I understand,
Is the rarest dish in all this land,
Which thus bedeck'd with a gay garland
Let us servire cantico.
Caput apri defero, etc.

Our steward hath provided this
In honor of the King of Bliss,
Which on this day to be served is
In Reginensi Atrio.
Caput apri defero,
etc., etc., etc.

The table was literally loaded with good cheer, and presented an epitome of country abundance, in this season of overflowing larders. A distinguished post was allotted to "ancient sirloin," as mine host termed it; being, as he added, "the standard of old English hospitality, and a joint of goodly presence, and full of expectation." There were several dishes quaintly decorated, and which had evidently something traditional in their embellishments; but about which, as I did not like to appear over-curious, I asked no questions.

I could not, however, but notice a pie, magnificently decorated with peacock's feathers, in imitation of the tail of that bird, which overshadowed a considerable tract of the table. This, the Squire confessed, with some little hesitation, was a pheasant-pie, though a peacock-pie was certainly the most authentical; but there had been such a mortality among the peacocks this season, that he could not prevail upon himself to have one killed. (Footnote: The peacock was anciently in great demand for stately entertainments. Sometimes it was made into a pie, at one end of which the head appeared above the crust in all its plumage, with the beak richly gilt; at the other end the tail was displayed. Such pies were served up at the solemn banquets of chivalry, when knights-errant pledged themselves to undertake any perilous enterprise, whence came the ancient oath, used by Justice Shalloy, "by cock and pie.")

The peacock was also an important dish for the Christmas feast; and Massinger, in his "City Madam," gives some idea of the extravagance with which this, as well as other dishes, was prepared for the gorgeous revels of the olden times:

"Men may talk of Country Christmasses,
"Their thirty pound butter'd eggs, their pies of carps' tongues;
"Their pheasants drench'd with ambergris; the carcases of three fat wethers bruised
for gravy to make sauce for a single peacock."

It would be tedious, perhaps, to my wiser readers, who may not have that foolish fondness for odd and obsolete things to which I am a little given, were I to mention the other makeshifts of this worthy old humorist, by which he was endeavoring to follow up, though at humble distance, the quaint customs of antiquity. I was pleased, however, to see the respect shown to his whims by his children and relatives; who, indeed, entered readily into the full spirit of them, and seemed all well versed in their parts; having doubtless been present at many a rehearsal. I was amused, too, at the air of profound gravity with which the butler and other servants executed the duties assigned them, however eccentric. They had an old-fashioned look; having, for the most part, been brought up in the household, and grown into keeping with the antiquated mansion, and the humors of its lord; and most probably looked upon all his whimsical regulations as the established laws of honorable housekeeping.

When the cloth was removed, the butler brought in a huge silver vessel of rare and curious workmanship, which he placed before the Squire. Its appearance was hailed with acclamation; being the Wassail Bowl, so renowned in Christmas festivity. The contents had been prepared by the Squire himself; for it was a beverage in the skillful mixture of which he particularly prided himself; alleging that it was too abstruse and complex for the comprehension of an ordinary servant. It was a potation, indeed, that might well make the heart of a toper leap within him; being composed of the richest and raciest wines, highly spiced and sweetened, with roasted apples bobbing about the surface. (Footnote: The Wassail Bowl was sometimes composed of ale instead of wine; with nutmeg, sugar, toast, ginger, and roasted crabs: in this way the nut-brown beverage is still prepared in some old families, and round the hearths of substantial farmers at Christmas.) It is also called Lamb's Wool, and is celebrated by Herrick in his "Twelfth Night":

> Next crowne the bowle full
> With gentle Lamb's Wool;
> Add sugar, nutmeg, and ginger,
> With store of ale too;
> And thus ye must doe
> To make the Wassaile a swinger.

The old gentleman's whole countenance beamed with a serene look of indwelling delight, as he stirred this mighty bowl. Having raised it to his lips, with a hearty wish of a merry Christmas to all present, he sent it brimming round the board, for every one to follow his example, according to the primitive style; pronouncing it "the ancient fountain of good feeling where all hearts met together." (Footnote: The custom of drinking out of the same cup gave place to each having his cup. When the steward came to the door with the Wassel, he was to cry three times, Wassel, Wassel, Wassel, and then the chappell (chaplain) was to answer with a song.—Archæologia.)

There was much laughing and rallying as the honest emblem of Christmas joviality circulated, and was kissed rather coyly by the ladies. When it reached Master Simon, he raised it in both hands, and with the air of a boon companion struck up an old Wassail chanson.

The brown bowle,
The merry brown bowle,
As it goes round about-a,
Fill
Still,
Let the world say what it will,
And drink your fill all out-a.

The deep canne,
The merry deep canne,
As thou dost freely quaff-a,
Sing
Fling,
Be as merry as a king,
And sound a lusty laugh-a. (Footnote: From Poor Robin's Almanac)

Much of the conversation during dinner turned upon family topics, to which I was a stranger. There was, however, a great deal of rallying of Master Simon about some gay widow, with whom he was accused of having a flirtation. This attack was commenced by the ladies; but it was continued throughout the dinner by the fat-headed old gentleman next to the parson, with the persevering assiduity of a slow hound; being one of those long-winded jokers, who, though rather dull at starting game, are unrivalled for their talents in hunting it down. At every pause in the general conversation, he renewed his bantering in pretty much the same terms; winking hard at me with both eyes, whenever he gave master Simon what he considered a home thrust. The latter, indeed, seemed fond of being teased on the subject, as old bachelors are apt to be; and he took occasion to inform me, in an undertone, that the lady in question was a prodigiously fine woman, and drove her own curricle.

The dinner-time passed away in this flow of innocent hilarity, and, though the old hall may have resounded in its time with many a scene of broader rout and revel, yet I doubt whether it ever witnessed more honest and genuine enjoyment. How easy it is for one benevolent being to diffuse pleasure around him; and how truly is a kind heart a fountain of gladness, making everything in its vicinity to freshen into smiles! The joyous disposition of the worthy Squire was perfectly contagious; he was happy himself, and disposed to make all the world happy; and the little eccentricities of his humor did but season, in a manner, the sweetness of this philanthropy.

When the ladies had retired, the conversation, as usual, became still more animated; many good things were broached which had been thought of during dinner, but which would not exactly do for a lady's ear; and though I cannot positively affirm that there was much wit uttered, yet I have certainly heard many contests of rare wit produce much less laughter. Wit, after all, is a mighty tart, pungent ingredient, and much too acid for some stomachs; but honest good-humor is the oil and wine of a merry meeting, and there is no jovial companionship equal to that where the jokes are rather small, and the laughter abundant.

The Squire told several long stories of early college pranks and adventures, in some of which the parson had been a sharer; though in looking at the latter, it required some effort of imagination to figure such a little dark anatomy of a man into the perpetrator of a madcap gambol. Indeed, the two college chums presented pictures of what men may be made by their different lots in life. The Squire had left the university to live lustily on his paternal domains, in the vigorous enjoyment of prosperity and sunshine, and had flourished on to a hearty and florid old age; whilst the poor parson, on the contrary, had dried and withered away among dusty tomes, in the silence and shadows of his study. Still there seemed to be a spark of almost extinguished fire, feebly glimmering in the bottom of his soul; and as the Squire hinted at a sly story of the parson and a pretty milkmaid, whom they once met on the banks of the Isis, the old gentleman made an "alphabet of faces," which, as far as I could decipher his physiognomy, I verily believe was indicative of laughter;—indeed, I have rarely met with an old gentleman that took absolute offense at the imputed gallantries of his youth.

I found the tide of wine and wassail fast gaining on the dry land of sober judgment. The company grew merrier and louder as their jokes grew duller. Master Simon was in as chirping a humor as a grasshopper filled with dew; his old songs grew of a warmer complexion, and he began to talk maudlin about the widow. He even gave a long song about the wooing of a widow which he informed me he had gathered from an excellent black-letter work, entitled "Cupid's Solicitor for Love," containing store of good advice for bachelors, and which he promised to lend me. The first verse was to this effect:—

> He that will woo a widow must not dally,
> He must make hay while the sun doth shine;
> He must not stand with her, shall I, shall I?
> But boldly say, Widow, thou must be mine.

This song inspired the fat-headed old gentleman, who made several attempts to tell a rather broad story out of Joe Miller, that was pat to the purpose; but he always stuck in the middle, everybody recollecting the latter part excepting himself. The parson, too, began to show the effects of good cheer, having gradually settled down into a doze, and his wig sitting most suspiciously on its side. Just at this juncture we were summoned to the drawing-room, and, I suspect, at the private instigation of mine host, whose joviality seemed always tempered with a proper love of decorum.

After the dinner-table was removed, the hall was given up to the younger members of the family, who, prompted to all kinds of noisy mirth by the Oxonian and Master Simon, made its old walls ring with their merriment, as they played at romping games. I delight in witnessing the gambols of children, and particularly at this happy holiday season, and could not help stealing out of the drawing-room on hearing one of their peals of laughter. I found them at the game of blindman's-buff. Master Simon, who was the leader of their revels, and seemed on all occasions to fulfil the office of that ancient Potentate, the Lord of Misrule, (Footnote: At Christmasse there was in the Kinge's house, wheresoever hee was lodged, a lorde of misrule, or mayster of merie disportes, and the like had ye in the house of every nobleman of hone, or good worshippe, were he spirtuall or temporall.—Stow) was blinded in the midst of the hall. The little beings were as busy about him as the mock fairies about Falstaff; pinching him, plucking at the skirts of his coat, and tickling him with straws. One fine blue-eyed girl of about thirteen, her flaxen hair all in beautiful confusion, her frolic face in a glow, her frock half torn off her shoulders, a complete picture of a romp, was the chief tormentor; and, from the slyness with which master Simon avoided the smaller game, and hemmed this wild little nymph in corners, and obliged her to jump shrieking over chairs, I suspected the rogue of being not a whit more blinded than was convenient.

When I returned to the drawing-room, I found the company seated round the fire, listening to the parson, who was deeply ensconced in a high-backed oaken chair, the work of some cunning artificer of yore, which had been brought from the library for his particular accommodation. From this venerable piece of furniture, with which his shadowy figure and dark weazen face so admirably accorded, he was dealing out strange accounts of the popular superstitions and legends of the surrounding country, with which he had become acquainted in the course of his antiquarian researches. I am half inclined to think that the old gentleman was himself somewhat tinctured with superstition, as men are very apt to be who live a recluse and studious life in a sequestered part of the country, and pore over black-letter tracts, so often filled with the marvelous and supernatural. He gave us several anecdotes of the fancies of the neighboring peasantry, concerning the effigy of the crusader, which lay on the tomb by the church-altar. As it was the only monument of the kind in that part of the country, it had always been regarded with feelings of superstition by the good wives of the village. It was said to get up from the tomb and walk the rounds of the churchyard in stormy nights, particularly when it thundered; and one old woman, whose cottage bordered on the churchyard, had seen it through the windows of the church, when the moon shone, slowly pacing up and down the aisles. It was the belief that some wrong had been left unredressed by the deceased, or some treasure hidden, which kept the spirit in a state of trouble and restlessness. Some talked of gold and jewels buried in the tomb, over which the specter kept watch; and there was a story current of a sexton in old times, who endeavored to break his way to the coffin at night, but, just as he reached it, received a violent blow from the marble hand of the effigy, which stretched him senseless on the pavement. These tales were often laughed at by some of the sturdier among the rustics, yet, when night came on, there were many of the stoutest unbelievers that were shy of venturing alone in the footpath that led across the churchyard.

From these and other anecdotes that followed, the crusader appeared to be the favorite hero of ghost-stories throughout the vicinity. His picture, which hung up in the hall, was thought by the servants to have something supernatural about it; for they remarked that, in whatever part of the hall you went, the eyes of the warrior were still fixed on you. The old porter's wife, too, at the lodge, who had been born and brought up in the family and was a great gossip among the maid-servants, affirmed, that in her young days she had often heard say, that on Midsummer eve, when it was well known all kinds of ghosts, goblins, and fairies become visible and walk abroad, the crusader used to mount his horse, come down from his picture, ride about the house, down the avenue, and so to the church to visit the tomb; on which occasion the church-door most civilly swung open of itself; not that he needed it, for he rode through closed gates and even stone walls, and had been seen by one of the dairy-maids to pass between two bars of the great park-gate, making himself as thin as a sheet of paper.

All these superstitions I found had been very much countenanced by the Squire, who, though not superstitious himself, was very fond of seeing others so. He listened to every goblin-tale of the neighboring gossips with infinite gravity, and held the porter's wife in high favor on account of her talent for the marvelous. He was himself a great reader of old legends and romances, and often lamented that he could not believe in them; for a superstitious person, he thought, must live in a kind of fairyland.

Whilst we were all attention to the parson's stories, our ears were suddenly assailed by a burst of heterogeneous sounds from the hall, in which were mingled something like the clang of rude minstrelsy, with the uproar of many small voices and girlish laughter. The door suddenly flew open, and a train came trooping into the room, that might almost have been mistaken for the breaking up of the court of Fairy. That indefatigable spirit, Master Simon, in the faithful discharge of his duties as Lord of Misrule, had conceived the idea of a Christmas mummery or masking; and having called in to his assistance the Oxonian and the young officer, who were equally ripe for anything that should occasion romping and merriment, they had carried it into instant effect. The old housekeeper had been consulted; the antique clothes-presses and wardrobes rummaged, and made to yield up the relics of finery that had not seen the light for several generations; the younger part of the company had been privately convened from the parlor and hall, and the whole had been bedizened out, into a burlesque imitation of an antique mask. (Footnote: Maskings or mummeries were favorite sports at Christmas in old times; and the wardrobes at halls and manor-houses were often laid under contribution to furnish dresses and fantastic disguisings. I strongly suspect Master Simon to have taken the idea of his from Ben Jonson's "Masque of Christmas.")

Master Simon led the van, as "Ancient Christmas," quaintly appareled in a ruff, a short cloak, which had very much the aspect of one of the old housekeeper's petticoats, and a hat that might have served for a village steeple, and must indubitably have figured in the days of the Covenanters. From under this his nose curved boldly forth, flushed with a frost-bitten bloom, that seemed the very trophy of a December blast. He was accompanied by the blue-eyed romp, dished up as "Dame Mince Pie," in the venerable magnificence of a faded brocade, long stomacher, peaked hat, and high-heeled shoes. The young officer appeared as Robin Hood, in a sporting dress of Kendal green, and a foraging cap with a gold tassel.

The costume, to be sure, did not bear testimony to deep research, and there was an evident eye to the picturesque, natural to a young gallant in the presence of his mistress. The fair Julia hung on his arm in a pretty rustic dress, as "Maid Marian." The rest of the train had been metamorphosed in various ways: the girls trussed up in the finery of the ancient belles of the Bracebridge line, and the striplings bewhiskered with burnt cork, and gravely clad in broad skirts, hanging sleeves, and full-bottomed wigs, to represent the character of Roast Beef, Plum Pudding, and other worthies celebrated in ancient maskings. The whole was under the control of the Oxonian, in the appropriate character of Misrule; and I observed that he exercised rather a mischievous sway with his wand over the smaller personages of the pageant.

The irruption of his motley crew, with beat of drum, according to ancient custom, was the consummation of uproar and merriment. Master Simon covered himself with glory by the stateliness with which, as Ancient Christmas, he walked a minuet with the peerless, though giggling, Dame Mince Pie. It was followed by a dance of all the characters, which, from its medley of costumes, seemed as though the old family portraits had skipped down from their frames to join in the sport. Different centuries were figuring at cross hands and right and left; the dark ages were cutting pirouettes and rigadoons; and the days of Queen Bess jigging merrily down the middle, through a line of succeeding generations.

The worthy Squire contemplated these fantastic sports, and this resurrection of his old wardrobe, with the simple relish of childish delight. He stood chuckling and rubbing his hands, and scarcely hearing a word the parson said, notwithstanding that the latter was discoursing most authentically on the ancient and stately dance at the Pavon, or peacock, from which he conceived the minuet to be derived. (Footnote: Sir John Hawkins, speaking of the dance called the Pavon, from pavo, a peacock, says: "It is a grave and majestic dance; the method of dancing it anciently was by gentlemen dressed with caps and swords, by those of the long robe in their gowns, by the peers in their mantles, and by the ladies in gowns with long trains, the motion whereof in dancing resembled that of a peacock."—History of Music) For my part, I was in a continual excitement from the varied scenes of whim and innocent gayety passing before me. It was inspiring to see wild-eyed frolic and warm-hearted hospitality breaking out from among the chills and glooms of winter, and old age throwing off his apathy, and catching once more the freshness of youthful enjoyment. I felt also an interest in the scene, from the consideration that these fleeting customs were posting fast into oblivion, and that this was, perhaps, the only family in England in which the whole of them was still punctiliously observed. There was a quaintness, too, mingled with all this revelry, that gave it a peculiar zest; it was suited to the time and place; and as the old manor-house almost reeled with mirth and wassail, it seemed echoing back the joviality of long departed years. (Footnote: At the time of the first publication of this paper, the picture of an old fashioned Christmas in the country was pronounced by some as out of date. The author had afterwards an opportunity of witnessing almost all the customs above described, existing in unexpected vigor in the skirts of Derbyshire and Yorkshire, where he passed the Christmas holidays. The reader will find some notice of them in the author's account of this sojourn at Newstead Abbey.)

But enough of Christmas and its gambols; it is time for me to pause in this garrulity. Methinks I hear the questions asked by my graver readers, "To what purpose is all this; how is the world to be made wiser by this talk?" Alas! is there not wisdom enough extant for the instruction of the world? And if not, are there not thousands of abler pens laboring for its improvement?—It is so much pleasanter to please than to instruct,—to play the companion rather than the preceptor.

What, after all, is the mite of wisdom that I could throw into the mass of knowledge; or how am I sure that my sagest deductions may be safe guides for the opinions of others? But in writing to amuse, if I fail, the only evil is in my own disappointment. If, however, I can by an lucky chance, in these days of evil, rub out one wrinkle from the brow of care, or beguile the heavy heart of one moment of sorrow; if I can now and then penetrate through the gathering film of misanthropy, prompt a benevolent view of human nature, and make my reader more in good-humor with his fellow-beings and himself, surely, surely, I shall not then have written entirely in vain.

From *The Sketch Book of Geoffrey Crayon, Gent.*, 1819.

Although Irving's friend, Dickens, is renowned today for his social commentary and tragic elements, The Pickwick Papers, *which gained him his first fame, initially made him the nineteenth-century Wodehouse. Here, drink conquers all.*

A Pleasant Day, with an Unpleasant Termination

Charles Dickens

The birds, who, happily for their own peace of mind and personal comfort, were in blissful ignorance of the preparations which had been making to astonish them, on the first of September, hailed it no doubt, as one of the pleasantest mornings they had seen that season. Many a young partridge who strutted complacently among the stubble, with all the finicking coxcombry of youth, and many an older one who watched his levity out of his little round eye, with the contemptuous air of a bird of wisdom and experience, alike unconscious of their approaching doom, basked in the fresh morning air with lively and blithesome feelings, and a few hours afterwards were laid low upon the earth. But we grow affecting; let us proceed.

In plain common-place matter-of-fact, then, it was a fine morning—so fine that you would scarcely have believed that the few months of an English summer had yet flown by. Hedges, fields, and trees, hill and moorland, presented to the eye, their ever-varying shades of deep rich green; scarce a leaf had fallen, scarce a sprinkle of yellow mingled with the hues of summer, warned you that autumn had begun. The sky was cloudless; the sun shone out bright and warm; the songs of birds, and hum of myriads of summer insects, filled the air; and the cottage gardens, crowded with flowers of every rich and beautiful tint, sparkled, in the heavy dew, like beds of glittering jewels. Everything bore the stamp of summer, and none of its beautiful colors had yet faded from the die.

Such was the morning, when an open carriage, in which were three Pickwickians (Mr. Snodgrass having preferred to remain at home), Mr. Wardle, and Mr. Trundle, with Sam Weller on the box beside the driver, pulled up by a gate at the road-side, before which stood a tall, raw-boned gamekeeper, and a half-booted, leather-legginned boy: each bearing a bag of capacious dimensions, and accompanied by a brace of pointers.

'I say,' whispered Mr. Winkle to Wardle, as the man let down the steps, 'they don't suppose we're going to kill game enough to fill those bags, do they?'

'Fill them!' exclaimed old Wardle. 'Bless you, yes! You shall fill one, and I the other; and when we've done with them, the pockets of our shooting-jackets will hold as much more.'

Mr. Winkle dismounted without saying anything in reply to this observation; but he thought within himself, that if the party remained in the open air, until he had filled one of the bags, they stood a considerable chance of catching colds in their heads.

'Hi, Juno, lass—hi, old girl; down, Daph, down,' said Wardle, caressing the dogs. 'Sir Geoffrey still in Scotland, of course, Martin?'

The tall gamekeeper replied in the affirmative, and looked with some surprise from Mr. Winkle, who was holding his gun as if he wished his coat pocket to save him the trouble of pulling the trigger, to Mr. Tupman, who was holding his as if he were afraid of it—as there is no earthly reason to doubt he really was.

'My friends are not much in the way of this sort of thing yet, Martin,' said Wardle, noticing the look. 'Live and learn, you know. They'll be good shots one of these days. I beg my friend Winkle's pardon, though; he has had some practice.'

Mr. Winkle smiled feebly over his blue neckerchief in acknowledgment of the compliment, and got himself so mysteriously entangled with his gun, in his modest confusion, that if the piece had been loaded, he must inevitably have shot himself dead upon the spot.

'You mustn't handle your piece in that ere way, when you come to have the charge in it, sir,' said the tall gamekeeper, gruffly, 'or I'm damned if you won't make cold meat of some on us.'

Mr. Winkle thus admonished abruptly altered its position and in so doing, contrived to bring the barrel into pretty sharp contact with Mr. Weller's head.

'Hallo!' said Sam, picking up his hat, which had been knocked off, and rubbing his temple. 'Hallo, sir! if you comes it this vay, you'll fill one o' them bags, and something to spare at one fire.'

Here the leather-legginned boy laughed very heartily, and then tried to look as if it was somebody else, wherat Mr. Winkle frowned majestically.

'Where did you tell the boy to meet us with the snack, Martin?' inquired Wardle.

'Side of One-tree Hill at twelve o'clock, sir.'

'That's not Sir Geoffrey's land, is it?'

'No, sir; but it's close by it. It's Captain Boldwig's land; but there'll be nobody to interrupt us, and there's a fine bit of turf there.'

'Very well,' said old Wardle. 'Now the sooner we're off the better. Will you join us at twelve, then Pickwick?'

Mr. Pickwick was particularly desirous to view the sport, the more especially as he was rather anxious in respect of Mr. Winkle's life and limbs. On so inviting a morning, too, it was very tantalizing to turn back, and leave his friends to enjoy themselves. It was, therefore with a very rueful air that he replied—

'Why, I suppose I must.'

'An't the gentleman a shot, sir?' inquired the long gamekeeper.

'No,' replied Wardle; 'and he's lame besides.'

'I should very much like to go,' said Mr. Pickwick, 'very much.'

There was a short pause of commiseration.

'There's a barrow t' other side the hedge,' said the boy. 'If the gentleman's servant would wheel along the paths, he could keep nigh us, and we could lift it over the stiles, and that.'

'The wery thing' said Mr. Weller, who was a party interested, inasmuch as he ardently longed to see the sport. 'The wery thing. Well said, smallcheck; I'll have it out in a minute.'

But here a difficulty arose. The long gamekeeper resolutely protested against the introduction into a shooting party, of a gentleman in a barrow, as a gross violation of all established rules and precedents.

It was a great objection, but not an insurmountable one. The gamekeeper having been coaxed and fed, and having, moreover, eased his mind by 'punching' the head of the inventive youth who had first suggested the use of the machine, Mr. Pickwick was placed in it, and off the party set; Wardle and the long gamekeeper leading the way, and Mr. Pickwick in the barrow propelled by Sam, bringing up the rear.

'Stop, Sam,' said Mr. Pickwick, when they had got half across the first field.

'What's the matter now?' said Wardle.

'I won't suffer this barrow to be moved another step,' said Mr. Pickwick, resolutely, 'unless Winkle carries that gun of his in a different manner.'

'How am I to carry it?' said the wretched Winkle.

'Carry it with the muzzle to the ground,' replied Mr. Pickwick.

'It's so unsportsman-like,' reasoned Winkle.

'I don't care whether it's unsportsman-like or not' replied Mr. Pickwick; 'I am not going to be shot in a wheelbarrow, for the sake of appearances, to please anybody.'

'I know the gentleman'll put that ere charge into somebody afore he's done,' growled the long man.

'Well, well—I don't mind,' said poor Winkle, turning his gunstock uppermost;—'there.'

'Anythin' for a quiet life,' said Mr. Weller; and on they went again.

'Stop!' said Mr. Pickwick, after they had gone a few yards further.

'What now?' said Wardle.

'That gun of Tupman's is not safe: I know it isn't,' said Mr. Pickwick.

'Eh? What! not safe?' said Mr. Tupman, in a tone of great alarm.

'Not as you are carrying it' said Mr. Pickwick. 'I am very sorry to make any further objection, but I cannot consent to go on, unless you carry it as Winkle does his.'

'I think you had better, sir,' said the long gamekeeper, 'or you're quite as likely to lodge the charge in yourself as in anything else.'

Mr. Tupman, with the most obliging haste, placed his piece in the position required, and the party moved on again; the two amateurs marching with reversed arms, like a couple of privates at a royal funeral.

The dogs suddenly came to a dead stop, and the party advancing stealthily a single pace, stopped too.

'What's the matter with the dogs' legs?' whispered Mr. Winkle. 'How queer they're standing.'

'Hush, can't you?' replied Wardle, softly. 'Don't you see, they're making a point?'

'Making a point!' said Mr. Winkle, staring about him, as if he expected to discover some particular beauty in the landscape which the sagacious animals were calling special attention to. 'Making a point! What are they pointing at?'

'Keep your eyes open,' said Wardle, not heeding the question in the excitement of the moment. 'Now then.'

There was a sharp whirring noise, that made Mr.Winkle start back as if he had been shot himself. Bang, bang, went a couple of guns—the smoke swept quickly away over the field, and curled into the air.

'Where are they?' said Mr. Winkle, in a state of the highest excitement, turning round and round in all directions. 'Where are they? Tell me when to fire. Where are they—where are they?'

'Where are they?' said Wardle, taking up a brace of birds which the dogs had deposited at his feet. 'Why, here they are.'

'No, no; I mean the others,' said the bewildered Winkle.

'Far enough off, by this time,' replied Wardle, coolly reloading his gun.

'We shall very likely be up with another covey in five minutes,' said the long gamekeeper. 'If the gentleman begins to fire now, perhaps he'll just get the shot out of the barrel by the time they rise.'

'Ha! ha! ha!' roared Mr. Weller.

'Sam,' said Mr. Pickwick, compassionating his follower's confusion and embarrassment.

'Sir.'

'Don't laugh.'

'Certainly not, sir.' So, by the way of indemnification, Mr. Well contorted his features from behind the wheelbarrow, for the exclusive amusement of the boy with the leggings, who thereupon burst into a boisterous laugh, and was summarily cuffed by the long gamekeeper, who wanted a pretext for turning round, to hide his own merriment.

'Bravo, old fellow!' said Wardle to Mr. Tupman; 'you fired that time, at all events.'

'Oh yes,' replied Mr. Tupman, with conscious pride. 'I let it off.'

'Well done. You'll hit something next time, if you look sharp. Very easy, ain't it?'

'Yes, it's very easy,' said Mr. Tupman. 'How it hurts one's shoulder, though. It nearly knocked me backwards. I had no idea these small fire-arms kicked so.'

'Ah,' said the old gentleman, smiling; 'you'll get used to it in time. Now then—all ready—all right with the barrow there?'

'All right, sir,' replied Mr. Weller.

'Come along, then.'

'Hold hard, sir,' said Sam, raising the barrow.

'Aye, aye,' replied Mr., Pickwick; and on they went, as briskly as need be.

'Keep that barrow back now,' cried Wardle, when it had been hoisted over a stile into another field, and Mr. Pickwick had been deposited in it once more.

'All right, sir,' replied Mr. Weller, pausing.

'Now, Winkle,' said the old gentleman, 'follow me softly, and don't be too late this time.'

'Never fear,' said Mr. Winkle. 'Are they pointing?'

'No, no; not now. Quietly now, quietly.' On they crept, and very quietly would have advanced, if Mr. Winkle, in the performance of some very intricate evolutions with his gun, had not accidently fired, at the most critical moment, over the boy's head, exactly in the very spot where the tall man's brain would have been, had he been there instead.

'Why, what on earth did you do that for?' said old Wardle, as the birds flew unharmed away.

'I never saw such a gun in my life,' replied poor Mr. Winkle, looking at the lock, as if that would do any good. 'It goes off on its own accord. It will do it.'

'Will do it!' echoed Wardle, with something of irritation in his manner. 'I wish it would kill something of its own accord.'

'It'll do that afore long, sir,' observed the tall man, in a low prophetic voice.

'What do you mean by that observation, sir?' inquired Mr. Winkle, angrily.

'Never mind, sir, never mind,' replied the long gamekeeper; 'I've no family myself, sir'; and this here boy's mother will get something handsome from Sir Geoffrey, if he's killed on his land. Load again, sir, load again.'

'Take away his gun,' cried Mr. Pickwick, from the barrow, horror-stricken at the long man's dark insinuations. 'Take away his gun, do you hear, somebody?'

Nobody, however, volunteered to obey the command; and Mr. Winkle, after darting a rebellious glance at Mr. Pickwick, reloaded his gun, and proceeded onwards with the rest.

We are bound, on the authority of Mr. Pickwick, to state, that Mr. Tupman's mode of proceeding evinced far more of prudence and deliberation, than that adopted by Mr. Winkle. Still, this by no means detracts from the great authority of the latter gentleman, on all matters connected with the field; because, as Mr. Pickwick beautifully observes, it has somehow or other happened, from time immemorial, that many of the best and ablest philosophers, who have been perfect lights of science in matters of theory, have been wholly unable to reduce them to practice.

Mr. Tupman's process, like many of our most sublime discoveries, was extremely simple. With the quickness and penetration of a man of genius, he had at once observed that the two great points to be attained were—first, to discharge his piece without injury to himself, and, secondly, to do so, without danger to the by-standers;—obviously, the best thing to do, after surmounting the difficulty of firing at all, was to shut his eyes firmly, and fire into the air.

On one occasion, after performing this feat, Mr. Tupman, on opening his eyes, beheld a plump partridge in the act of falling wounded to the ground. He was on the point of congratulating Mr. Wardle on his invariable success, when the gentleman advanced towards him, and grasped him warmly by the hand.

'Tupman,' said the old gentleman, 'you singled out that particular bird?'

'No,' said Mr. Tupman—'no.'

'You did,' said Wardle. 'I saw you do it—I observed you pick him out—I noticed you, as you raised your piece to take aim; and I will say this, that the best shot in existence could not have done it more beautifully. You are an older hand at this, than I thought you, Tupman; you have been out before.'

It was in vain for Mr. Tupman to protest, with a smile of self-denial, that he never had. The very smile was taken as evidence to the contrary; and from that time forth, his reputation was established. It is not the only reputation that has been acquired as easily, nor are such fortunate circumstances confined to partridge-shooting.

Meanwhile, Mr. Winkle flashed and blazed, and smoked away, without producing any material results worthy of being noted down; sometimes expending his charge in mid-air, and at others sending it skimming along so near the surface of the ground as to place the lives of the two dogs on a rather uncertain and precarious tenure. As a display of fancy shooting, it was extremely varied and curious; as an exhibition of firing with any precise object, it was upon the whole, perhaps a failure. It is an established axiom, that 'every bullet has its billet.' If it apply in an equal degree to shot, those of Mr. Winkle were unfortunate foundlings, deprived of their natural rights, cast loose upon the world, and billeted nowhere.

'Well,' said Wardle, walking up the side of the barrow, and wiping the streams of perspiration from his jolly red face; 'smoking day, isn't it?'

'It is, indeed,' replied Mr. Pickwick. 'The sun is tremendously hot, even to me. I don't know how you must feel it.'

'Why,' said the old gentleman, 'pretty hot. It's past twelve, though. You see that green hill there?'

'Certainly.'

'That's the place where we are to lunch; and by Jove, there's the boy with the basket, punctual as clock-work!'

'So he is,' said Mr. Pickwick, brightening up. 'Good boy that. I'll give him a shilling presently. Now, then, Sam, wheel away.'

'Hold on, sir, said Mr. Weller, invigorated with the prospect of refreshments. 'Out of the vay, young leathers. If you walley my precious life, don't upset me as the gen'l'm'n said to the driver when they was carryin' him to Tyburn.' And quickening his pace to a sharp run, Mr. Weller wheeled his master nimbly to the green hill, shot him dexterously out by the very side of the basket, and proceeded to unpack it with the utmost despatch.

'Weal pie,' said Mr. Weller, soliloquizing, as he arranged the eatables on the grass. 'Wery good thing is weal pie, when you know the lady as made it, and is quite sure it an't kittens; and arter all, though where's the odds, when they're so like weal that the wery piemen themselves don't know the difference?'

'Don't they, Sam?' said Mr. Pickwick.

'Not they, sir,' replied Mr. Weller, touching his hat. 'I lodged in the same house vith a pieman once, sir, and a wery nice man he was—reg'lar clever chap, too—make pies out o' anything, he could. "What a number o' cats you keep, Mr. Brooks" says I, when I'd got intimate with him. "Ah," says he, "I do—a good many," says he. "You must be wery fond o' cats," says I. "Other people is," says he, a winkin' at me; "they an't in season till the winter, though," says he. "Not in season!" says I. "No," says he, "fruits is in, cats is out." "Why, what do you mean?" says I. "Mean?" says he. "That I'll never be a party to the combination o' butchers, to keep up the prices o' meat," says he. "Mr. Weller," says he, a squeezing my hand wery hard, and vispering in my ear—"don't mention this here agin—but it's the seasonin' as does it. They're all made o' them noble animals," says he, a pointin' to a wery nice little tabby kitten, "and I seasons 'em for beefsteak, weal, or kidney, 'cordin' to the demand. And more than that," says he, "I can make a weal a beef-steak, or a beef-steak a kidney, or any one on 'em a mutton, at a minute's notice, just as the market changes, and appetites wary!"'

'He must have been a very ingenious young man, that, Sam,' said Mr. Pickwick, with a slight shudder.

'Just was, sir,' replied Mr. Weller, continuing his occupation of emptying the basket, 'and the pies was beautiful. Tongue; well that's a wery good thing when it an't a woman's. Bread—knuckle o' ham, reg'lar picter—cold beef in slices, wery good. What's in them stone jars, young touch-and-go?'

'Beer in this one,' replied the boy, taking from his shoulder a couple of large stone bottles, fastened together by a leathern strap—'cold punch in t' other.'

'And a wery good notion of a lunch it is, take it altogether,' said Mr. Weller, surveying his arrangement of the repast with great satisfaction. 'Now, gen'l'm'n, "fall on," as the English said to the French when they fixed bagginets.'

It needed no second invitation to induce the party to yield full justice to the meal; and as little pressing did it require to induce Mr. Weller, the long gamekeeper, and the two boys, to station themselves on the grass, at a little distance, and do good execution upon a decent proportion of the viands. An old oak afforded a pleasant shelter to the group, and a rich prospect of arable and meadow land, intersected with luxuriant hedges, and richly ornamented with wood, lay spread out below them.

'This is delightful—thoroughly delightful!' said Mr. Pickwick, the skin of whose expressive countenance was rapidly peeling off, with exposure to the sun.

'So it is: so it is, old fellow,' replied Wardle. 'Come; a glass of punch!'

'With great pleasure,' said Mr. Pickwick; the satisfaction of whose countenance, after drinking it, bore testimony to the sincerity of the reply.

'Good,' said Mr. Pickwick, smacking his lips. 'Very good. I'll take another. Cool; very cool. Come, gentlemen,' continued Mr. Pickwick, still retaining his hold upon the jar, 'a toast. Our friends at Dingley Dell.'

The toast was drunk with loud acclamations.

'I'll tell you what I shall do, to get up my shooting again,' said Mr. Winkle, who was eating bread and ham with a pocket-knife. 'I'll put a stuffed partridge on the top of a post, and practice at it, beginning at a short distance, and lengthening it by degrees. I understand it's capital practice.'

'I know a gen'l'm'n, sir,' said Mr. Weller, 'as did that, and begun at two yards; but he never tried it on agin; for he blowed the bird right clean away at the first fire, and nobody ever seed a feather on him arterwards.'

'Sam,' said Mr. Pickwick.

'Sir,' replied Mr. Weller.

'Have the goodness to reserve your anecdotes till they are called for.'

'Cert'nly, sir.'

Here Mr. Weller winked the eye which was not concealed by the beer-can he was raising to his lips with such exquisiteness, that the two boys went into spontaneous convulsions, and even the long man condescended to smile.

'Well, that certainly is most capital cold punch,' said Mr. Pickwick, looking earnestly at the stone bottle; 'and the day is extremely warm, and—Tupman, my dear friend, a glass of punch?'

'With the greatest delight,' replied Mr. Tupman; and having drank that glass, Mr. Pickwick took another, just to see whether there was any orange peel in the punch, because orange peel always disagreed with him, and finding that there was not, Mr.

Pickwick took another glass to the health of their absent friend, and then felt himself imperatively called upon to propose another in honour of the punch-compounder, unknown.

This constant succession of glasses produced considerable effect upon Mr. Pickwick, his countenance beamed with the most sunny smiles, laughter played around his lips, and good-humoured merriment twinkled in his eye. Yielding by degrees to the influence of the exciting liquid, rendered more so by the heat, Mr. Pickwick expressed a strong desire to recollect a song which he had heard in his infancy, and the attempt proving abortive, sought to stimulate his memory with more glasses of punch, which appeared to have quite a contrary effect; for, from forgetting the words of the song, he began to forget how to articulate any words at all; and finally, after rising to his legs to address the company in an eloquent speech, he fell into the barrow, and fast asleep, simultaneously.

The basket having been repacked and it being found perfectly impossible to awaken Mr. Pickwick from his torpor, some discussion took place whether it would be better for Mr. Weller to wheel his master back again, or to leave him where he was, until, they should all be ready to return. The latter course was at length decided on; and as the further expedition was not to exceed an hour's duration, and as Mr. Weller begged very hard to be one of the party, it was determined to leave Mr. Pickwick asleep in the barrow, and to call for him on their return. So away they went, leaving Mr. Pickwick snoring most comfortably in the shade.

That Mr. Pickwick would have continued to snore in the shade until his friends came back, or, in default thereof, until the shades of evening had fallen on the landscape, there appears no reasonable cause to doubt; always supposing that he had been suffered to remain there in peace. But he was not suffered to remain there in peace. And this was what prevented him.

Captain Boldwig was a fierce little man in a stiff black neckerchief and blue surtout, who, when he did condescend to walk about his property, did it in company with a thick rattan stick with a brass ferrule, and a gardener and sub-gardener with meek faces, to whom (the gardeners, not the stick) Captain Boldwig gave his orders with all due grandeur and ferocity: for Captain Boldwig's wife's sister had married a Marquis, and the Captain's house was a villa, and his lands 'grounds,' and it was all very high, and mighty, and great.

Mr. Pickwick had not been asleep half an hour when little Captain Boldwig, followed by the two gardeners, came striding along as fast as his size and importance would let him; and when he came near the oak tree, Captain Boldwig paused, and drew a long breath, and looked at the prospect as if he thought the prospect ought to be highly gratified at having him to take notice of it; and then he struck the ground emphatically with his stick, and summoned the head gardener.

'Hunt,' said Captain Boldwig.

'Yes, sir,' said the gardener.

'Roll this place to-morrow morning—do you hear, Hunt?'

'Yes, sir.'

'And remind me to have a board done about trespassers, and spring guns, and all that sort of thing, to keep the common people out. Do you hear Hunt; do you hear?'

'I'll not forget it, sir.'

'I beg your pardon, sir,' said the other man, advancing, with his hand to his hat.

'Well, Wilkins, what's the matter with you?' said Captain Boldwig.

'I beg your pardon, sir—but I think there have been trespassers here to-day.'

'Ha!' said the Captain, scowling around him.

'Yes, sir—they have been dining here, I think, sir.'

'Why, confound their audacity, so they have,' said Captain Boldwig, as the crumbs and fragments that were strewn upon the grass met his eye. 'They have actually been devouring their food here. I wish I had the vagabonds here!' said the Captain, clenching the thick stick.

'I wish I had the vagabonds here!' said the Captain, wrathfully.

'Beg your pardon, sir,' said Wilkins, 'but—'

'But what? Eh?' roared the Captain; and following the timid glance of Wilkins, his eyes encountered the wheelbarrow and Mr. Pickwick.

'Who are you, you rascal?' said the Captain, administering several pokes to Mr. Pickwick's body with the thick stick. 'What's your name?'

'Cold punch,' murmured Mr. Pickwick, as he sunk to sleep again.

'What?' demanded Captain Boldwig.

No reply.

'What did he say his name was?' asked the Captain.

'Punch, I think, sir,' replied Wilkins.

'That's his impudence, that's his confounded impudence,' said Captain Boldwig. 'He's only feigning to be asleep now,' said the Captain, in a high passion. 'He's drunk; he's a drunken plebian. Wheel him away, Wilkins, wheel him away directly.'

'Where shall I wheel him to, sir?' inquired Wilkins with great timidity.

'Wheel him to the Devil,' replied Captain Boldwig.

'Very well, sir,' said Wilkins.

'Stay,' said the Captain.

Wilkins stopped accordingly.

'Wheel him,' said the Captain, 'wheel him to the Pound; and let us see whether he calls himself Punch when he comes to himself. He shall not bully me, he shall not bully me. Wheel him away.'

Away Mr. Pickwick was wheeled in compliance with this imperious mandate; and the great Captain Boldwig, swelling with indignation, proceeded on his walk.

Inexpressible was the astonishment of the little party when they returned, to find that Mr. Pickwick had disappeared, and taken the wheelbarrow with him. It was the most mysterious and unaccountable thing that was ever heard of. For a lame man to have go upon his legs without any previous notice, and walked off, would have been most extraordinary; but when it came to his wheeling a heavy barrow before him, by way of amusement, it grew positively miraculous. They searched every nook and corner round, together and separately; they shouted, whistled, laughed, called—and all with the same result. Mr. Pickwick was not to be found. After some hours of fruitless search, they arrived at the unwelcome conclusion that they must go home without him.

Meanwhile Mr. Pickwick had been wheeled to the Pound, and safely deposited therein, fast asleep in the wheelbarrow, to the immeasurable delight and satisfaction, not only of all the boys in the village, but three-fourths of the whole population, who had gathered round, in expectation of his waking. If their most intense gratification had been excited by seeing him wheeled in, how many hundredfold was their joy increased when, after a few indistinct cries of 'Sam!' he sat up in the barrow, and gazed with indescribable astonishment on the faces before him.

A general shout was of course the signal of his having woke up; and his involuntary inquiry of 'What's the matter?' occasioned another, louder than the first, if possible.

'Here's a game!' roared the populace.

'Where am I?' exclaimed Mr. Pickwick.

'In the Pound,' replied the mob.

'How came I here? What was I doing? Where was I brought from?'

'Boldwig! Captain Boldwig!' was the only reply.

'Let me out,' cried Mr. Pickwick. 'Where's my servant? Where are my friends?'

'You ain't got no friends. Hurrah!' Then there came a turnip, then a potato, and then an egg: with a few other little tokens of the playful disposition of the many-headed.

How long this scene might have lasted, or how much Mr. Pickwick might have suffered, no one can tell, had not a carriage, which was driving swiftly by, suddenly pulled up, from whence there descended old Wardle and Sam Weller, the former of whom, in far less time than it takes to write it, if not to read it, had made his way to Mr. Pickwick's side, and placed him in the vehicle, just as the latter had concluded the third and last round of a single combat with the town-beadle.

'Run to the Justice's!' cried a dozen voices.

'Ah, run avay,' said Mr. Weller, jumping up on the box. 'Give my compliments—Mr. Veller's compliments—to the Justice, and tell him I've spiled his beadle, and that, if he'll swear in a new 'un, I'll come back agin to-morrow and spile him. Drive on, old feller.'

'I'll give directions for the commencement of an action for false imprisonment against this Captain Boldwig, directly I get to London,' said Mr. Pickwick, as soon as the carriage turned out of the town.

'We were trespassing, it seems,' said Wardle.

'I don't care,' said Mr. Pickwick, 'I'll bring the action.'

'No you won't,' said Wardle.

'I will by—' but as there was a humorous expression in Wardle's face, Mr. Pickwick checked himself, and said, 'Why not?'

'Because,' said old Wardle, half-bursting with laughter, 'because they might turn round on some of us, and say we had taken too much cold punch.'

Do what he would, a smile would come into Mr. Pickwick's face; the smile extended into a laugh; the laugh into a roar; the roar became general. So, to keep up their good humour, they stopped at the first roadside tavern they came to, and ordered a glass of brandy-and-water all round, with a magnum of extra strength for Mr. Samuel Weller.

From *The Pickwick Papers*, Charles Dickens. Contains all the copyright emendations made in the text as revised by the author in 1867 and 1868. Books, Inc., pp. 235–248.

Absinthe was a great inspiration to many European and Louisianan writers of the late nineteenth century. Made of anise and wormwood, its slightly hallucinogenic and aphrodisiac qualities led it to be outlawed in most countries; this occurred in the United States in 1911. It has become, however, popular again in early twenty-first-century London, where drinking it is seen as a sign of opposition to Tony Blair and "New Labour." Your editor drinks it whenever he is in the Metropolis.

With Flowers and with Women

Charles Cros

With Flowers, and with Women,
With Absinthe, and with this Fire,
We can divert ourselves a while,
Act out our part in some drama.

Absinthe, on a winter evening,
Lights up in green the sooty soul;
And Flowers, on the beloved,
Grow fragrant before the clear Fire.

Later, kisses lose their charm
Having lasted several seasons;
And after mutual betrayals
We part one day without a tear.

We burn letters and bouquets.
And fire takes our bower;
And if sad life is salvaged
Still there is Absinthe and its hiccups. . . .

The portraits are eaten by flames. . . .
Shrivelled fingers tremble. . . .

We die from sleeping long
With Flowers, and with Women.

 A step back in time—a trip to the Twilight Zone.
—RANDY BARBATA, BARBATA'S STEAK HOUSE, 20001 VENTURA BOULEVARD,
WOODLAND HILLS, CALIFORNIA

Mark Twain is considered to be one of the best, if not the best of American writers. In this selection, this quintessential American encounters foreign drunkenness—to his own advantage.

The Usefulness of Getting Drunk

Mark Twain

We made the tramp from Martigny to Argentiére in eight hours. We beat all the mules and wagons; we didn't usually do that. We hired a sort of open baggage-wagon for the trip down the valley to Chamonix, and then devoted an hour to dining. This gave the driver time to get drunk. He had a friend with him, and this friend also had time to get drunk.

When we drove off, the driver said all the tourists had arrived and gone by while we were at dinner: "but," said he, impressively, "be not disturbed that—remain tranquil—give yourselves no uneasiness—their dust rises far before us, you shall see it fade and disappear far behind us—rest you tranquil, leave all to me—I am the king of drivers. Behold!"

Down came his whip, and away we clattered. I never had such a shaking up in my life. The recent flooding rains had washed the road clear away in places, but we never slowed down for anything. We tore right along, over rocks, rubbish, gullies, open fields—sometimes with one or two wheels on the ground, but generally with none. Every now and then that calm, good-natured madman would bend a majestic look over his shoulder at us and say, "Ah, you perceive? It is as I have said—I am the king of drivers." Every time we just missed going to destruction, he would say, with tranquil happiness, "Enjoy it, gentlemen, it is very rare, it is very unusual—it is given to few to ride with the king of drivers—and observe, it is as I have said, *I* am he."

He spoke in French, and punctuated with hiccoughs. His friend was French, too, but spoke in German—using the same system of punctuation, however. The friend called himself the "Captain of Mont Blanc," and wanted us to make the ascent with him. He said he had made more ascents than any other man,—forty-seven,—and his brother had made thirty-seven. His brother was the best guide in the world, except himself—but he, yes, observe him well,—he was the "Captain of Mont Blanc"—the title belonged to none other.

The "king" was as good as his word—he overtook that long procession of tourists and went by it like a hurricane. The result was that we got choicer rooms at the hotel in Chamonix than we should have done if his majesty had been a slower artist—or rather, if he hadn't most providentially got drunk before he left Argentiére.

From *A Tramp Abroad,* 1904. New York and London: Harper and Brothers, pp. 183–185.

G. K. Chesterton is most renowned as an apologist for Catholicism and as a superb paradox-revealer. In the following essay, he makes a plea for the common man's right to wine.

Wine When It Is Red

G. K. Chesterton

I suppose that there will be some wigs on the green in connection with the recent manifesto signed by a string of very eminent doctors on the subject of what is called "alcohol." "Alcohol" is, to judge by the sound of it, an Arabic word, like "algebra" and "Alhambra," those two other unpleasant things. The Alhambra in Spain I have never seen; I am told that it is a low and rambling building; I allude to the far more digni- fied erection in Leicester Square. If it is true, as I surmise, that "alcohol" is a word of the Arabs, it is interesting to realize that our general word for the essence of wine and beer and such things comes from a people which has made particular war against them. I suppose that some aged Moslem chieftain sat one day at the opening of his tent and, brooding with black brows and cursing in his black beard over wine as the symbol of Christianity, racked his brains for some word ugly enough to express his racial and religious antipathy, and suddenly spat out the horrible word "alcohol." The fact that the doctors had to use this word for the sake of scientific clearness was really a great disadvantage to them in fairly discussing the matter. For the word really involves one of those beggings of the question which makes these moral matters so difficult. It is quite a mistake to suppose that when a man desires an alcoholic drink, he necessarily desires alcohol.

Let a man walk ten miles steadily on a hot summer's day along a dusty English road, and he will soon discover why beer was invented. The fact that beer has a very slight stimulating quality will be quite among the smallest reasons that induce him to ask for it. In short, he will not be in the least desiring alcohol; he will be desiring beer. But, of course, the question cannot be settled in such a simple way. The real difficulty which confronts everybody, and which especially confronts doctors, is that the extra- ordinary position of man in the physical universe makes it practically impossible to treat him in either one direction or the other in a purely physical way. Man is an exception, whatever else he is. If he is not the image of God, then he is a disease of the dust. If it is not true that divine being fell, then we can only say that one of the animals went entirely off its head. In neither case can we really argue very much from the body of man simply considered as the body of an innocent and healthy animal. His body has got much mixed up with his soul, as we see in the supreme issue of sex. It may be worth while uttering the warning to wealthy philanthropists and idealists that this argument from the animal should not be thoughtlessly used, even against the atrocious evils of excess; it is an argument that proves too little or too much. Doubtless, it is unnatural to be drunk. But then in a real sense it is unnatural to be human. Doubtless the intemperate workman wastes his tissues in drinking; but no one knows how much the sober workman wastes his tissues in working. No one knows how much the wealthy philanthropist wastes his tissues by talking; or in much rare conditions, by thinking. All the human things are more dangerous than anything that affects the beasts—sex, poetry, property, religion. The real case against drunkenness is not that it calls up the beast, but that it calls up the Devil. It does not call up the beast, and if it did it would not matter much as a rule; the beast is a harmless and rather amiable creature, as anybody can see by watching cattle. There is nothing bestial about intoxication; and certainly there is nothing intoxicating or even particularly lively about beasts. Man is always something worse or something better than an animal; and a mere argument from animal perfection never touches him at all. Thus, in sex no animal is either chivalrous or obscene. And no animal ever invented anything so bad as drunkenness—or so good as drink.

The pronouncement of these particular doctors is very clear and uncompromising; in the modern atmosphere, indeed, it even deserves some credit for moral courage. The majority of modern people, of course, will probably agree with it in so far as it declares that alcoholic drinks are often of supreme value in emergencies of illness; but many people, I fear, will open their eyes at the emphatic terms in which they describe such drink as considered as a beverage; but they are not content with declaring that drinking in moderation is harmless: they distinctly declare that it is in moderation beneficial. But I fancy that, in saying this, the doctors had in mind a truth that runs somewhat counter to the common opinion. I fancy that it is the experience of most doctors that giving any alcohol for sickness (though often necessary) is about the most morally dangerous way of giving it. Instead of giving it to a healthy person who has many other forms of life, you are giving it to a desperate person, to whom it is the only form of life. The invalid can hardly be blamed if by some accident of his erratic and overwrought condition he comes to remember the thing as the very water of vitality and to use it as such. For in so far as drinking is really a sin it is not because drinking is wild, but because drinking is tame; not in so far as it is anarchy, but in so far as it is slavery. Probably the worst way to drink is to drink medicinally. Certainly the safest way to drink is to drink carelessly; that is, without caring much for anything, and especially not caring for the drink.

The doctor, of course, ought to be able to do a great deal in the way of restraining those individual cases where there is plainly an evil thirst; and beyond that the only hope would seem to be in some increase, or rather, some concentration of ordinary public opinion on the subject. I have always held consistently my own modest theory on the subject. I believe that if by some method the local public-house could be as definite and isolated a place as the local post-office or the local railway station, if all types of people passed through it for all types of refreshment, you would have the same safeguard against a man behaving in a disgusting way in a tavern that you have against his behaving in a disgusting way in a post-office: simply the presence of his ordinary sensible neighbors. In such a place the kind of lunatic who wants to drink an unlimited number of whiskies would be treated with the same severity with which the post office authorities would treat an amiable lunatic who had an appetite for licking an unlimited number of stamps. It is a small matter whether in either case a technical refusal would be officially employed. It is an essential matter that in both cases the authorities could rapidly communicate with friends and family of the mentally afflicted person. At least, the postmistress would not dangle a strip of tempting sixpenny stamps before the enthusiast's eyes as he was being dragged away with his tongue out. If we made drinking open and official we might be taking one step towards making it careless. In such things to be careless is to be sane: for neither drunkards nor Moslems can be careless about drink.

From *All Things Considered*, 1908. London: Methuen and Company, pp. 231–236.

As with his close friend Chesterton, Hilaire Belloc had a reputation for tippling. In fact, it was said of the two that they had misread the Nicene Creed and thought it proclaimed belief in "One, Holy, Catholic, and Alcoholic *Church."*

On Port

Hilaire Belloc

I had already set this title down long ago for a meditation when a sacred fear seized me, for I knew that I was approaching holy ground. I return to it now reluctantly not with temerity but with awe and trembling. Port is an adopted son of England, and anyone who attacks him is attacking the family—a formidable enterprise. Anyone who praises him may by some slight overpraise or misjudges praise give even more offense than by open attack. It is always so with family things: better keep out of them.

Of foreign things which are also modern (meaning by modern that which we came to know after the renewal of England in the seventeenth century) Port comes earlier than Tea, and it seems to me at least to have a nobler lineage, for it is of Christendom, whereas Tea is of Cathay. The name of the town, Oporto, means no more than "the port," and when they talked of Oporto wine and then shortened it into Port they were getting back to the English form of the Latin word for harbor, which English form had come in its turn from the French form of the Latin word *Portus,* as one should say a "he-door," just as *Porta* is a "she-door." A port was the gate into and out of a country. That, if I remember aright, was one of the arguments in favor of the Crown during the violent quarrels of King and Parliament before the Civil Wars. I will not risk my memory upon the occasion of the quarrel when this argument turned up. I seem to remember it was Bates' Case. But anyhow the reasoning was that the King had a right to say what should come in and out of the country by its ports because the ports were the gates of the kingdom, and a man could not be master in his own house unless he had control of the doors thereof. So here you have the word "port" come home again in quite a different sense, and used to represent quite a different thing from what it had done till those few generations ago.

When a man said, "I hope to make port," everyone up to a certain date knew what he meant; he could only mean one thing; it was a sentence that could only have been spoken at sea or in prospect of a sea voyage. But after that date a man saying, "I hope to make port," might mean one of two totally different things. He might mean, "I hope to reach harbor," or he might mean, "I hope by the use of chemicals to produce something sufficiently like portwine to deceive the vulgar."

You could not have two phrases with more dissimilar meanings! And all because the old word "port" having taken a long circular flight came to roost again on another branch.

It is so with many another word, "stuff," for instance, and "rout"; and a delight it is (to me at least) to follow verbal gyrations and transformations of that kind. "Stuff" began with the wad of tow or whatnot which was soaked in oil and stuck into the narrow necks of great jars to prevent the wine going sour. Then it wandered about and came to mean "cloth," and then "matter," then it branched off and hooked arms with "nonsense"; then it turned into a verb and meant filling. It hasn't done yet. It still has far to go and many a summerset to turn.

As for "rout," it came from "déroute," which meant being driven off your "route" or road, and that word "route" comes according to the learned Wiener from the Assyrian for a postal system. But I am getting tired of all this digression, and I must make for Port again.

Though I know nothing essential of Port (and that is why I am writing on it), yet I have, like the rest of my fellow citizens, a certain empiric or experimental knowledge with it. I have drunk a glass of it from time to time, and I have seen strange things happen in connection with it. For instance, a friend of mine (it is now forty years ago) said to me, as he pulled the cork out of a bottle, "I have here some very remarkable port which came from my grandfather; it is of the year so-and-so" (mentioning a date before the flood), "and I have kept it specially for this occasion." I thanked him as in duty bound. Then with the gesture and expression of one performing a high religious rite he let loose imprisoned Bacchus from his spongy door. But on the appearance of the god, the god had changed complexion and had even changed his very nature. For in color he came out like dirty milk, and in taste like nothing on earth. My friend said, " it has passed its prime." Anyhow, there is no doubt that this Port, as Port, had ceased to function. It was "defunct" in the fullest and most absolute sense of the term.

Then, also, I have been given as Port under alien stars something which was about as much like Port as rice rolled in blacking is like caviar. This strange foreign Port which has appeared before me like an evil vision in town after town, from Cracow to Canyon City, has always turned up in a new garment of its own. It has always borne some hitherto quite unknown, and to me, fantastic label. But that does not only apply to Port, that matter of labels, and it works both ways, I mean an absurd label may be attached to an exceedingly good bottle of wine.

I have an example of this in my memory, when, in the first year of the Great War, a hostess asked me whether I would tell her what I thought of a certain wine. She brought this wine. It was a white wine and bore a label on which was printed the simple words *Mes Amours*. I confessed that the vintage was unfamiliar to me, as was the label, which was surrounded by a lot of little dancing Cupids linked together by a ribbon. But when I came to drink this wine it was a really good Montrachet. Now how did a really good Montrachet get into a bottle with a label like that? I cannot tell you. It is one of the myriad mysteries with which we are surrounded from the cradle to the grave; and as for any man who denies mystery, let him be anathema; and a donkey to boot.

I have far from exhausted (I am not quite sure if these last five words are good English), anyhow I am far from having exhausted my superficial and very provincial acquaintance with Port, but I will squeeze in one last tale about it here. A deservedly famous conoozer of Claret, *jam senex* (the conoozer, not the wine) was offered some Port by a much younger man and when he had tasted it was asked what he thought of it. He answered, "it's all alcohol to me!"

With this immortal phrase I leave you. I am not sure that I have not printed that story before, but it is worth printing thousands of times and distributing throughout the human race.

"Drinking is a good thing for everybody—if you enjoy."
—RAMON CASTANEDA, OWNER, *H.M.S. BOUNTY*, 3357 WILSHIRE BOULEVARD
LOS ANGELES, CALIFORNIA

From *The Silence of the Sea*, 1940. New York: Sheed and Ward, pp. 219–223.

We make a great leap into the twentieth century, into the America of the Roaring '20s. Fitzgerald was the literary expression of the time, whose irrepressible spirit could find no better outlet than the speakeasies. It was a mad time, created by the insanity of Prohibition.

Mr. In and Mr. Out

F. Scott Fitzgerald

Mr. In and Mr. Out are not listed by the census-taker. You will search for them in vain through the social register or the births, marriages, and deaths, or the grocer's credit list. Oblivion has swallowed them and the testimony that they ever existed at all is vague and shadowy, and inadmissible in a court of law. Yet I have it upon the best authority that for a brief space Mr. In and Mr. Out lived, breathed, answered to their names and radiated vivid personalities of their own.

During the brief span of their lives they walked in their native garments down the great highway of a great nation; were laughed at, sworn at, chased, and fled from. Then they passed and were heard of no more.

They were already taking form dimly, when a taxicab with the top open breezed down Broadway in the faintest glimmer of May dawn. In this car sat the souls of Mr. In and Mr. Out discussing with amazement the blue light that had so precipitately colored the sky behind the statue of Christopher Columbus, discussing with bewilderment the old, gray faces of the early risers which skimmed palely along the street like blown bits of paper on a gray lake. They were agreed on all things, from the absurdity of the bouncer in Childs' to the absurdity of the business of life. They were dizzy with the extreme maudlin happiness that the morning had awakened in their glowing souls. Indeed, so fresh and vigorous was their pleasure in living that they felt it should be expressed by loud cries.

"Ye-ow-ow!" hooted Peter, making a megaphone with his hands—and Dean joined in with a call that, though equally significant and symbolic, derived its resonance from its very inarticulateness.

"Yo-ho! Yea! Yoho! Yo-buba!"

Fifty-third Street was a bus with a dark, bobbed-hair beauty atop; Fifty-second was a street cleaner who dodged, escaped, and sent up a yell of, "Look where you're aimin'!" in a pained and grieved voice. At Fiftieth Street a group of men on a very white sidewalk in front of a very white building turned to stare after them, and shouted:

"Some party, boys!"

At Forty-ninth Street Peter turned to Dean. "Beautiful morning," he said gravely, squinting up his owlish eyes.

"Probably is."

"Go get some breakfast, hey?"

Dean agreed—with additions.

"Breakfast and liquor."

"Breakfast and liquor," repeated Peter, and they looked at each other, nodding. "That's logical."

Then they both burst into loud laughter.

"Breakfast and liquor! Oh, gosh!"

"No such thing," announced Peter.

"Don't serve it? Ne'mind. We force 'em serve it. Bring pressure bear."

"Bring pressure bear."

The taxi cut suddenly off Broadway, sailed along a cross street, and stopped in front of a heavy tomb-like building in Fifth Avenue.

"What's idea?"

The taxi-driver informed them that this was Delmonico's.

This was somewhat puzzling. They were forced to devote several minutes to intense concentration, for if such an order had been given there must have been a reason for it.

"Somep'm 'bouta coat," suggested the taxi-man.

That was it. Peter's overcoat and hat. He had left them at Delmonico's. Having decided this, they disembarked from the taxi and strolled toward the entrance arm in arm.

"Hey!" said the taxi-driver.

"Huh?"

"You better pay me."

They shook their heads in shocked negation.

"Later, not now—we give orders, you wait."

65

The taxi-driver objected; he wanted his money now. With the scornful conde-scension of men exercising tremendous self-control they paid him.

Inside Peter groped in vain through a dim, deserted check-room in search of his coat and derby.

"Gone, I guess. Somebody stole it."

"Some Sheff student."

"All probability."

"Never mind," said Dean, nobly. "I'll leave mine here too—then we'll both be dressed the same."

He removed his overcoat and hat and was hanging them up when his roving glance was caught and held magnetically by two large squares of cardboard tacked to the two coat-room doors. The one on the left-hand door bore the word "In" in big black letters, and the one on the right-hand door flaunted the equally emphatic word "Out."

"Look!" he exclaimed happily—

Peter's eyes followed his pointing finger.

"What?"

"Look at the signs. Let's take 'em."

"Good idea."

"Probably pair very rare an' valuable signs. Probably come in handy."

Peter removed the left-hand sign from the door and endeavored to conceal it about his person. The sign being of considerable proportions, this was a matter of some difficulty. An idea flung itself at him, and with an air of dignified mystery he turned his back. After an instant he wheeled dramatically around, and stretching out his arms displayed himself to the admiring Dean. He had inserted the sign in his vest, completely covering his shirt front. In effect, the word "in" had been painted upon his shirt in large black letters.

"Yoho!" cheered Dean. "Mister In."

He inserted his own sign in like manner.

"Mister Out!" he announced triumphantly. "Mr. In meet Mr. Out."

They advanced and shook hands. Again laughter overcame them and they rocked in a shaken spasm of mirth.

"Yoho!"

"We probably get a flock of breakfast."

"We'll go—go to the Commodore."

Arm in arm they sallied out the door, and turning east on Forty-fourth Street set out for the Commodore.

As they came out a short dark soldier, very pale and tired, who had been wandering listlessly along the sidewalk, turned to look at them.

He started over as though to address them, but as they immediately bent on him glances of withering unrecognition, he waited until they had started unsteadily down the street, and then followed at about forty paces, chuckling to himself and saying "Oh, boy!" over and over under his breath, in delighted, anticipatory tones.

Mr. In and Mr. Out were meanwhile exchanging pleasantries concerning their future plans.

"We want liquor; we want breakfast. Neither without the other. One and indivisible."

"We want both 'em!"

"Both 'em!"

It was quite light now, and passers-by began to bend curious eyes on the pair. Obviously they were engaged in a discussion, which afforded each of them intense amusement, for occasionally a fit of laughter would seize upon them so violently that, still with their arms interlocked, they would bend nearly double.

Reaching the Commodore, they exchanged a few spicy epigrams with the sleepy-eyed doorman, navigated the revolving door with some difficulty, and then made their way through a thinly populated but startled lobby to the dining-room, where a puzzled waiter showed them an obscure table in a corner. They studied the bill of fare helplessly, telling over the items to each other in puzzled mumbles.

"Don't see any liquor here," said Peter reproachfully.

The waiter became audible but unintelligible.

"Repeat," continued Peter, with patient tolerance, "that there seems to be unexplained and quite distasteful lack of liquor upon bill of fare."

"Here!" said Dean confidently, "let me handle him." He turned to the waiter— "Bring us—bring us—" he scanned the bill of fare anxiously. "Bring us a quart of champagne and a—a—probably ham sandwich."

The waiter looked doubtful.

"Bring it!" roared Mr. In and Mr. Out in chorus.

The waiter coughed and disappeared. There was a short wait during which they were subjected without their knowledge to a careful scrutiny by the headwaiter. Then the champagne arrived, and at the sight of it Mr. In and Mr. Out became jubilant.

"Imagine their objecting to us having champagne for breakfast—jus' imagine."

They both concentrated upon the vision of such an awesome possibility but the feat was too much for them. It was impossible for their joint imaginations to conjure up a world where any one might object to any one else having champagne for breakfast. The waiter drew the cork with an enormous pop—and their glasses immediately foamed with pale yellow froth.

"Here's health, Mr. In."

"Here's same to you, Mr. Out."

The waiter withdrew; the minutes passed; the champagne became low in the bottle.

"It's—it's mortifying," said Dean suddenly.

"Wha's mortifying?"

"The idea their objecting us having champagne breakfast."

"Mortifying?" Peter considered. "yes, tha's word—mortifying."

Again they collapsed into laughter, howled, swayed, rocked back and forth in their chairs, repeating the word "mortifying" over and over to each other—each repetition seeming to make it only more brilliantly absurd.

After a few more gorgeous minutes they decided on another quart. Their anxious waiter consulted his immediate superior, and this discreet person gave implicit instructions that no more champagne should be served. Their check was brought.

Five minutes later, arm in arm, they left the Commodore and made their way through a curious, staring crowd along Forty-second Street, and up Vanderbilt Avenue to the Biltmore. There, with sudden cunning, they rose to the occasion and traversed the lobby, walking fast and standing unnaturally erect.

Once in the dining-room they repeated their performance. They were torn between intermittent convulsive laughter and sudden spasmodic discussions of politics, college, and the sunny state of their dispositions. Their watches told them that it was now nine o'clock, and a dim idea was born in them that they were on a memorable party, something that they would remember always. They lingered over the second bottle. Either of them had only to mention the word "mortifying" to send them both into riotous gasps. The dining-room was whirring and shifting now; a curious lightness permeated and rarefied the heavy air.

They paid their check and walked out into the lobby.

It was at this moment that the exterior doors revolved for the thousandth time that morning, and admitted into the lobby a very pale young beauty with dark circles under her eyes, attired in a much-rumpled evening dress. She was accompanied by a plain stout man, obviously not an appropriate escort.

At the top of the stairs this couple encountered Mr. In and Mr. Out.

"Edith," began Mr. In, stepping toward her hilariously and making a sweeping bow, "darling, good morning."

The stout man glanced questioningly at Edith, as if merely asking her permission to throw this man summarily out of the way.

" 'Scuse familiarity," added Peter, as an afterthought. "Edith, good-morning."

He seized Dean's elbow and impelled him into the foreground.

"Meet Mr. In, Edith, my bes' frien'. Inseparable. Mr. In and Mr. Out."

Mr. Out advanced and bowed; in fact, he advanced so far and bowed so low that he tipped slightly forward and only kept his balance by placing a hand lightly on Edith's shoulder.

"I'm Mr. Out, Edith," he mumbled pleasantly, "S'misterin Misterout."

" 'Smisterinandout," said Peter proudly.

But Edith stared straight by them, her eyes fixed on some infinite speck in the gallery above her. She nodded slightly to the stout man, who advanced bull-like and with a sturdy brisk gesture pushed Mr. In and Mr. Out to either side. Through this alley he and Edith walked.

But ten paces farther on Edith stopped again—stopped and pointed to a short, dark soldier who was eyeing the crowd in general, and the tableau of Mr. In and Mr. Out in particular, with a sort of puzzled, spell-bound awe.

"There," cried Edith. "See there!"

Her voice rose, became somewhat shrill. Her pointing finger shook slightly.

"There's the soldier who broke my brother's leg."

There were a dozen exclamations; a man in a cutaway coat left his place near the desk and advanced alertly; the stout person made a sort of lightning-like spring toward the short, dark soldier, and then the lobby closed around the little group and blotted them from the sight of Mr. In and Mr. Out.

But to Mr. In and Mr. Out this event was merely a particolored iridescent segment of a whirring, spinning world.

They heard loud voices; they saw the stout man spring; the picture suddenly blurred.

Then they were in an elevator bound skyward.

"What floor, please?" said the elevator man.

69

"Any floor," said Mr. In.

"Top floor," said Mr. Out.

"This is the top floor," said the elevator man.

"Have another floor put on," said Mr. Out.

"Higher," said Mr. In.

"Heaven," said Mr. Out.

From "May Day" © 1920 by Smart Set Company, Inc., *The Short Stories of F. Scott Fitzgerald,* edited and with a new preface by Matthew J. Bruccoli, 1989. New York: Charles Scribner's Sons, pp. 135–140.

Better known for his chilling tales of horror, Arthur Machen was an extremely good host and very fun-loving. Given to strong political, social, and religious opinions, he was contemptuous of the anti-alcohol crowd. Hence the following essay.

Six Dozen of Port

Arthur Machen

Many good people must have been sadly shocked to read of a certain recent bequest which has been recorded in the papers. The testator, a wealthy solicitor, directed his executors to buy six dozen of the best vintage port for the benefit of "his good friend and partner," Mr. Blank, in the hope that in drinking it Mr. Blank would be reminded of cordial relations that had existed between them for many years.

I can imagine, as I say, that horror of varying degrees of intensity will be aroused by these dispositions. There are all the people who hate life, who have many names and styles and titles. They call themselves intellectuals, or, sometimes, the intelligentsia; I suppose because they have no intelligent understanding or perception of anything whatever. When you talk to them about literature they will be cross with you if you suggest that the thing exists or has ever existed outside Russia—always excepting, of course, one or two honored and "conscientious" English names. If you talk to them about education, they will laugh at anything except physical science out of court, reserving always psychoanalysis, which turns the whole world of waking and dreaming into a peculiarly putrid and silly form of nightmare nastiness. But the real mark of this sect is their hatred of life. That is a large order, you will say. So it is. But a lady of my acquaintance put the matter very clearly once before one of the most distinguished members of the sect, a gentleman who never touches good meat or good drink and thinks the habit of smoking a disgusting vice. The lady had been listening to the Intellectual for some time, and then she turned and said: "I tell you what, George. What would do you good would be to be brought to bed with twins; then you might know something about life!" The lady was proceeding *per impossibile*, of course; but I think one sees her point. The sect in question argues most acutely against this and that and the other, and argues so well that you are confounded by the strength of its position—till you perceive that what they object to is not this or that or the other, but life itself, and, indeed, life is full of objectionable incidents; but it is all the life we know anything about.

Need I say that to the intellectuals this bequest of six dozen of the very best port will be highly offensive? They are not all teetotalers, perhaps, but they would be agreed to holding port to be at best a very trivial thing. I remember one of them being highly irritated by one of the most savory volumes of modern times, Professor Saintsbury's *Notes from a Cellar Book,* to read which is almost—but not quite—as rare a treat as the drinking of the choice and curious delicacies in wine that it describes. "A record of a state of things which has fortunately quite passed away"; in these words, or in words to that effect, did the Intellectual describe the golden volume of one who is learned, it is true, in wine, but learned also in the literatures of the world, a true Professor of the humaner letters. These people, with certain exceptions, always speak with scorn of the Classics. If we get beaten in a foreign market, if the current goes wrong on "the Met.," if anything happens that ought not to happen, they say that it is because our educational system is all wrong, since we teach our boys Latin and Greek instead of physical science. Consequently, as despisers of what the Irish hedge school-master called "the Haythen mysthology," these people know nothing about the story of Dionysos, the Wine God; how he went all over the world, civilizing the nations by teaching them the culture of the vine, and they have not heard the moral fable of King Pentheus, who resisted the civilizing mission of Dionysos, tried to keep the vine out of his kingdom, and, as a natural consequence, went mad and came to a dreadful end, being in fact torn to pieces. This sounds nonsense, doesn't it? But it has just been happening in our own day. Russia went dry—and then Russia went mad and Bolshevist; and even our advanced "thinkers" are coming to the conclusion that Bolshevism is a very dreadful end indeed. Russia has been torn to pieces. As for the United States of America, a distinguished American statesman has declared recently that the increase of crime in the States since the coming of Prohibition has been terrific and terrifying.

And, by the way, I have been reading lately about two recent enactments of the Legislature of the Sovereign Commonwealths of Kentucky and Georgia. Kentucky has declared that Evolution is contrary to the laws of the State: Georgia enacts that the man who goes out fishing without his wife's leave is a felon, and that the punishment of his crime shall be a sentence of five years' penal servitude. As I was saying, Pentheus was very odd in his manner towards the end.

But, as I say, the Intellectual is by no means always a teetotaler. His position is rather that meat and drink are matters of no importance, that they are unworthy of the consideration of a sage, and that a man who thinks much of his dinner and his glass of vintage port is an inferior person who thinks of meat and drink because he has no mind to think of anything higher. That is why the intelligentsia dislike Dickens, who loves nothing better than to describe a feast and the joys of good eating and good drinking. "This is an inferior mind," they say. "If you would see true greatness read Luntic Kolnyatsch in the original Gibrisch"—with Mr. Max Beerbohm's leave. "He specializes in skin-disease, vermin, and suicide, subjects fit for the genius of the modern world." All I can say is that it strikes me as a very strange frame of mind. You have something like it in the seventeenth-century Puritans who hated a great number of noble and beautiful and goodly things; you have, perhaps, the original of it all in the fifth-century Manichees who founded their faith on a logical basis, at all events. They were persuaded that the world with all that therein is was made by the devil, and therefore that everything in the world was very evil. A really thoroughgoing Manichee could not break a crust of bread without uttering a long apology for doing so, which was his grace before meat. This was all very well and consistent; but the intelligentsia have no very fervid belief in the devil; so why do they either hate or, at least, despise old vintage port and, in general, all the good things of life? Remember the "Kreutzer Sonata" by Tolstoi, the ancestor of the whole family of Kolnyatsch. Here you have a book which strikes not at this detail or that; not at the bottle of old port, or the good cigar, or the roast partridge, but at the very source of all life. It is thoroughgoing, certainly, for if the "Kreutzer Sonata" doctrine were carried out we should be delivered from all our troubles, since there would soon be none of us left. Tolstoi held, as it seems, that no children should be born into the world; presumably, therefore, he held that existence in itself is an evil, thus approximating to the doctrine of Buddhism. Well, Buddhism is of India, and Manes, the founder of the Manichees, was a Persian: the East has always been inclined to teetotalism; that is, to the denial of the joy of life.

You will remember, of course, that highly popular best seller "Rasselas," by the late Samuel Johnson, L.L.D. Rasselas, Prince of Abyssinia, is speaking:

"By what means," said the Prince, "are the Europeans thus powerful; or why, since they can so easily visit Asia and Africa for trade and conquest, cannot the Asiaticks and Africans invade their coasts, plant colonies in their ports, and give laws to their natural princes? The same wind that carries them back would bring us thither."

The puzzle is addressed to the sage, Imlac, the prince's philosophic counselor. Imlac, with some circumlocution, gives it up, and Johnson himself, commenting on the passage many years after, did the same. He said that he could see no real explanation of the remarkable facts.

The explanation is, of course, easy enough. The East, as I said, has always been inclined to teetotalism, with all that is implied in that term.

Let us be warned in time. Woe to us if we take to despising good drink while the myriads of millions of China take to strong ale and vintage port. Our day will be done. "Mene Mene" will be written on the wall. Let us rather honor the memory and imitate the example of the good man of Gray's Inn, who left six dozen bottles of the finest port to his old friend. I am sure that he was a good man. If a man talks to me of the sacred cause of Humanity, I lock up my few silver spoons. If he speaks of Liberty, I know that he has a Bill in his pocket by which it will be made penal to out of bed after ten P.M. But he who speaks well of port is, as the Greeks said of their best men, beautiful and good.

From *Dog and Duck*, Arthur Machen, 1924. New York: Alfred A. Knopf, pp. 168–175.

Yet another star of the roaring '20s, Mencken excoriated the United States as "a Commonwealth of third-rate minds." Certainly, Prohibition—the topic of this essay— might be seen as justifying his views to some extent. Doubtless today he would be certain that we had improved—unless of course he were to encounter California's prohibition of smoking in bars.

The Noble Experiment

H. L. Mencken

Prohibition went into effect on January 16, 1920, and blew up at last on December 5, 1933—an elapsed time of twelve years, ten months, and nineteen days. It seemed almost a geological epoch while it was going on, and the human suffering that it entailed must have been a fair match for that of the Black Death or the Thirty Years' War, but I should say at once that my own share of the blood, sweat and tears was extremely meagre. I was, so far as I have been able to discover, the first man south of the Mason and Dixon line to brew a drinkable home-brew, and as a result my native Baltimore smelled powerfully of malt and hops during the whole horror, for I did not keep my art to myself, but imparted it to anyone who could be trusted—which meant anyone save a few abandoned Methodists, Baptists and Presbyterians, most of them already far gone in glycosuria, cholelithiasis or gastrohydrorrhea, and all of them soon so low in mind and body that they could be ignored.

My seminary was run on a sort of chain-letter plan. That is to say, I took ten pupils, and then each of the ten took ten, and so on *ad infinitum*. There were dull dogs in Baltimore who went through the course forty or fifty times, under as many different holders of my degrees, and even then never got beyond a nauseous *Malzsuppe,* fit only for policemen and Sunday-school superintendents. But there were others of a much more shining talent, and I put in a great deal of my time in 1921 and 1922 visiting their laboratories, to pass judgment on their brews. They received me with all the deference due to a master, and I was greatly bucked up by their attentions. In fact, those attentions probably saved me from melancholia, for during the whole of the twelve years, ten months and nineteen days I was a magazine editor, and a magazine editor is a man who lives on a sort of spiritual Bataan, with bombs of odium taking him incessantly from the front and torpedoes of obloquy harrying him astern.

But I would not have you think that I was anything like dependent, in that abominable time, upon home-brew, or that I got down any really formidable amount of it. To be sure, I had to apply my critical powers to many thousands of specimens, but I always took them in small doses, and was careful to blow away a good deal of the substance with the foam. The home-brew, when drinkable at all, was a striking proof of the indomitable spirit of man, but in the average case it was not much more. Whenever the mood to drink purely voluptuously was on me I preferred, of course, the product of professional brewmasters, and, having been born lucky, I usually found it. Its provenance, in those days, was kept a kind of military secret, but now that the nightmare is over and jails no longer yawn I do not hesitate to say that, in so far as my own supply went, most of it came from the two lowermost tiers of Pennsylvania counties. Dotted over that smiling pastoral landscape there were groups of small breweries that managed successfully, by means that we need not go into, to stall off the Prohibition agents, and I had the privilege and honor of getting down many a carboy of their excellent product both in Baltimore, where I lived, and in New York, where I had my office.

When I say New York I mean the city in its largest sense—the whole metropolitan region. As a matter of fact, the malt liquor on tap on the actual island of Manhattan was usually bad, and often downright poisonous. When I yearned for a quaff of the real stuff I went to Union Hill, N.J., and if not to Union Hill, then to Hoboken. Both of these great outposts radiated a bouquet of malt and hops almost as pungent as Baltimore's, and in Union Hill there was a beer-house that sticks in my memory as the most comfortable I have ever encountered on this earth. Its beers were perfect, its victuals were cheap and nourishing, its chairs were designed by osteological engineers specializing in the structure of the human pelvis, and its waiters, Axel, Otto, Julius and Raymond, were experts at their science. This incomparable dump was discovered by the late Philip Goodman, then transiently a theatrical manager on Broadway and all his life a fervent beer-drinker, and he and I visited it every time I was in New York, which was pretty often. We would ease into our canons' stalls in the early evening and continue in residence until Axel, Otto, Julius and Raymond began to snore in their corner and the colored maintenance engineer, Willie, turned his fire-hose into the washroom. Then back by taxi to Weehawken, from Weehawken to

Forty-second street by the six-minute ferry, and from Forty-second street by taxi again to the quick, lordly sleep of quiet minds and pure hearts.

The fact that the brews on tap in that Elysium came from lower Pennsylvania naturally suggested an expedition to the place of their origin, and Goodman and I laid many plans for making the trip in his car. But every time we started out we dropped in on Axel, Otto, Julius and Raymond for stirrup cups, and that was as far as we ever got. Alone, however, I once visited Harrisburg on newspaper business, and there had the felicity of drinking close to the *Urquell.* That was in the primitive days when New York still bristled with peepholes and it was impossible to get into a strange place without a letter from a judge, but in Harrisburg there were no formalities. I simply approached a traffic cop and asked him where reliable stuff was to be had. "Do you see that kaif there?" he replied, pointing to the corner. "Well, just go in and lay down your money. If you don't like it, come back and I'll give you another one." I liked it well enough, and did not trouble him further.

I should add, however, that I once came so near going dry in Pennsylvania, and in the very midst of a huge fleet of illicit breweries, that the memory of it still makes me shiver. This was at Bethlehem in the Lehigh Valley, in 1924. I had gone to the place with my publisher, Alfred Knopf, to hear the celebrated Bach Choir, and we were astounded after the first day's sessions to discover that not a drop of malt liquor was to be had in the local pubs. This seemed strange and unfriendly, for it is well known to every musicologist that the divine music of old Johann Sebastian cannot be digested without the aid of its natural solvent. But so far as we could make out there was absolutely none on tap in the Lehigh Valley, though we searched high and low, and threw ourselves upon the mercy of cops, taxi-drivers, hotel clerks, the Elks, the rev. clergy, and half the tenors and basses of the choir. All reported that Prohibition agents had been sighted in the mountains a few days before, and that as a result hundreds of kegs had been buried and every bartender was on the alert. How we got through the second day's sessions I don't know; the music was magnificent, but our tonsils became so parched that we could barely join in the final Amen. Half an hour before our train was scheduled to leave for New York we decided to go down to the Lehigh station and telegraph to a bootician in the big city, desiring him to start westward at once and meet us at Paterson, N.J. On the way to the station we discussed this madcap scheme dismally, and the taxi-driver overheard us. He was a compassionate man, and his heart bled for us.

"Gents," he said, "I hate to horn in on what ain't none of my business, but if you feel that bad about it I think I know where some stuff is to be had. The point is, can you get it?"

We at once offered him money to introduce us, but he waved us off.

"It wouldn't do you no good," he said. "These Pennsylvania Dutch never trust a hackman."

"But where is the place?" we breathed.

"I'm taking you to it," he replied, and in a moment we were there.

It was a huge, blank building that looked like a forsaken warehouse, but over a door that appeared to be tightly locked there was the telltale sign, "Sea Food"—the universal euphemism for beerhouse in Maryland and Pennsylvania throughout the thirteen awful years. We rapped on the door and presently it opened about half an inch, revealing an eye and part of a mouth. The ensuing dialogue was *sotto voce* but *staccato* and *appassionata*. The eye saw that we were famished, but the mouth hesitated.

"How do I know," it asked, "that you ain't two of them agents?"

The insinuation made us boil, but we had to be polite.

"*Agents!*" hissed Knopf. "What an idea! Can't you *see* us? Take a good look at us."

The eye looked, but the mouth made no reply.

"Can't you tell musicians when you see them?" I broke in. "Where did you ever see a Prohibition agent who looked so innocent, so moony, so dumb? We are actually fanatics. We came here to hear Bach. Is this the way Bethlehem treats its guests? We came a thousand miles, and now—"

"*Three* thousand miles," corrected Knopf.

"*Five* thousand," I added, making it round numbers.

Suddenly I bethought me that the piano score of the B minor mass had been under my arm all the while. What better introduction? What more persuasive proof of our *bona fides*? I held up the score and pointed to the title on the cover. The eye read:

J. S. Bach
Mass in B Minor

The eye flicked for an instant or two, and then the mouth spoke. "Come in, gents," it said. As the door opened our natural momentum carried us into the bar in one leap, and there we were presently immersed in two immense *Humpen*. The quality we did not pause to observe; what we mainly recalled later was the astounding modesty of the bill, which was sixty-five cents for five *Humpen*—Knopf had two and I had three—and two sandwiches. We made our train just as it was pulling out.

It was a narrow escape from death in the desert, and we do not forget all these years afterward that we owed it to Johann Sebastian Bach, that highly talented and entirely respectable man, and especially to his mass in B minor. In the great city of Cleveland, Ohio, a few months later, I had much worse luck. I went there, in my capacity of newspaper reporter, to help cover the Republican national convention which nominated Calvin Coolidge, and I assumed like everyone else that the Prohibition agents would lay off while the job was put through, if only as a mark of respect to their commander-in-chief. This assumption turned out to be erroneous. The agents actually clamped down on Cleveland with the utmost ferocity, and produced a drought that was virtually complete. Even the local cops and newspaper reporters were dry, and many of the latter spent a large part of their time touring the quarters of the out-of-town correspondents, begging for succor. But the supplies brought in by the correspondents were gone in a few days, and by the time the convention actually opened a glass of malt liquor was as hard to come by in Cleveland as an honest politician.

The news of this horror quickly got about, and one morning I received a dispatch in cipher from a Christian friend in Detroit, saying that he was loading a motor-launch with ten cases of bottled beer and ale, and sending it down the Detroit river and across Lake Erie in charge of two of his goons. They were instructed, he said, to notify me the instant they arrived off the Cleveland breakwater. Their notice reached me the next afternoon, but by that time the boys were nominating Cal, so I could not keep the rendezvous myself, but had to send an agent. This agent was Paul de Kruif, then a young man of thirty-four, studying the literary art under my counsel. Paul was a fellow of high principles and worthy of every confidence; moreover, he was dying of thirst himself. I started him out in a rowboat, and he was gone three hours. When he got back he was pale and trembling, and I could see at a glance that some calamity had befallen. When he got his breath he gasped out the story.

The two goons, it appeared, had broken into their cargo on the way down from Detroit, for the weather was extremely hot. By the time they anchored off the Cleveland breakwater they had got down three cases, and while they were waiting for de Kruif they knocked off two more. This left but five—and they figured that it was just enough to get them back to Detroit, for the way was uphill all the way, as a glance at a map will show. De Kruif, who was a huge and sturdy Dutchman with a neck like John L. Sullivan, protested violently and even undertook to throw them overboard and priate the launch and cargo, but they pulled firearms on him, and the best he could do was to get six bottles. These he drank on his return in the rowboat, for the heat, as I have said, was extreme. As a result, I got nothing whatsoever; indeed, not a drop of malt touched my throat until the next night at 11:57, when the express for Washington and points East crossed the frontier of the Maryland Free State.

This was my worst adventure during Prohibition, and in many ways it remains the worst adventure of my whole life, though I have been shot at four times and my travels have taken me to Albania, Trans-Jordan and Arkansas. In Maryland, there was always plenty, and when I was in New York Goodman and I made many voyages to Union Hill. One hot night in 1927, while we were lolling in the perfect beerhouse that I have mentioned, a small but excellent band was in attendance, and we learned on inquiry that it belonged to a trans-Atlantic liner of foreign registry, then berthed at one of the North river docks. Through Axel and Raymond we got acquainted with the leader, and he told us that if we cared to accompany him and his men back to the ship they would set up some real Pilsner. We naturally accepted, and at five o'clock the next morning we were still down in the stewards' dining-room on H-deck, pouring in *Seidel* after *Seidel* and victualing royally on black bread and *Leberwurst*. The stewards were scrupulous fellows and would not bootleg, but Goodman had some talent for mathematics, and it was not hard for him to figure out a tip that would cover what we had drunk of their rations, with a reasonable *Zuschlag* added.

Thereafter, we visited that lovely ship every time it was in port, which was about once every five weeks, and in a little while we began to add other ships of the same and allied lines, until in the end we had a whole fleet of them, and had access to Pilsner about three weeks out of four, and not only to Pilsner but also to Munchner, Dortmunder, Wurzburger and Kulmbacher. It was a long hoof down the dark pier to the cargo port we had to use, and a long climb from the water-line down to H-deck, but we got used to the exertion and even came to welcome it, for we were both under medical advice to take more exercise. When we went aboard, usually at 10 or 11 P.M., there was no one on the dock save a customs watchman sitting on a stool at the street entrance, chewing tobacco, and when we debarked at 4 or 5 A.M. the same watchman was still there, usually sound asleep.

Gradually, such being the enticements of sin, we fell into the habit of sneaking a couple of jugs past the watchman—most often, of Germany brandy, or *Branntwein.* It was abominable stuff, but nevertheless it was the real McCoy, and Goodman and I found it very useful—he for drugging his actors and I for dishing out to the poets who infested my magazine office. One night there was some sort of celebration aboard ship—as I recall it, the birthday of Martin Luther—and the stewards put on a special spread. The *pièce de résistance* was a *Wurst* of some strange but very toothsome kind, and Goodman and I got down large rashers of it, and praised it in high, astounding terms. The stewards were so pleased by our appreciation that they gave us two whole ones as we left, and so we marched up the pier to the street, each with a bottle of *Branntwein* in one coat pocket and a large, globulous sausage in the other. To our surprise we found the customs watchman awake. More, he halted us.

"What have you got there in your pockets?" he demanded.

We turned them out, and he passed over the two bottles without a word, but the sausages set him off to an amazing snorting and baying.

"God damn me," he roared, "if I ever seen the like. Ain't you got *no sense whatever?* Here I try to be nice to you, and let you get something 100% safe in your system, and what do you hand me? What you hand me is that you try to do some *smuggling* on me. Yes, *smuggling.* I know the law and so do you. If I wanted to turn you in I could send you to Atlanta for the rest of your life. God damn if I ain't *ashamed* of you."

With that he grabbed the two sausages and hugged them to him. Goodman and I, conscious of guilt, stood silent, with flushed faces and downcast eyes. What was there to say? Nothing that we could think of. We had been taken red-handed in a deliberate violation of the just laws of this great Republic. We had tried with malice prepense to rob the Treasury of the duty on two valuable sausages—say, 67½ cents at 25% *ad valorem* on a valuation of $2.50 for the pair. The amount, to be sure, was small, but the principle was precious beyond price. In brief, we were common felons, dirt criminals, enemies to society, and as reprehensible, almost, as so many burglars, hijackers or Prohibition agents.

The watchman howled on for two or three minutes, seeking, apparently, to impress upon us the heinousness of our offense. We needed no such exposition. Our consciences were devouring us with red-hot fangs. There was no need for us to say a word, for we radiated repentance and regret. But finally, as the watchman dismissed us with a parting blast, Goodman ventured upon a question.

"Do you," he asked, "want the bottles too?"

"Hell, no," replied the watchman. "What *I* am trying to bust up is *smuggling*."

 James Joyce, John Steinbeck, Jack Kerouac—a drink at Chumley's makes them live again!
—BRITTA STEINER, WAITRESS, CHUMLEY'S (EST. 1926), 86 BEDFORD STREET, NEW YORK CITY

From *A Choice of Days* by H. L. Mencken © 1980 by H. L. Mencken Estate, "Heathen Days, 1890–1936," 1943. New York: Alfred A. Knopf, pp. 307–320.

*Since the eighteenth century, the French have had a reputation as wine worshippers.
In this selection, Colette shows us just how true this is!*

The Lucky Hour of Great Wines

Colette

I was very well brought up. As a convincing proof of such a categorical assertion, let me say that when I was barely three years of age my father, who believed in gentle and progressive methods, gave me a full liqueur glass of a reddish-brown wine sent to him from his native Southern France; the Muscat Wine of Frontignan.

It was like a sun-stroke, or love at first sight, or the sudden realization of a nervous system; this consecration rendered me a worthy disciple of wine for ever afterwards. A little later, I learnt to quaff my glass of mulled wine, aromatic, with cinnamon and lemon, to a dinner of boiled chestnuts. At the age when one can barely read I was spelling out, drop by drop, red Burgundies, old and light, and dazzling Yquems. Champagne passed in its turn, a murmur of foam, leaping pearls of air, across birthday dinners and first communion festivities: with it came gray Puissaye truffles . . . a fine lesson from which I acquired familiar and discreet knowledge of wine, not swallowed greedily, but measured out into narrow glasses, absorbed in mouthfuls with long spaces in between, and carefully reflected upon.

It was between my eleventh and my fifteenth years that this beautiful educational program was completed. My mother feared that, as I grew older, I should become anemic. One by one, she unearthed from their dry sand some bottles which were aging beneath our house in a cellar—it is, thank Heavens!, still intact—carved out of the granite itself. Whenever I think about it, I envy the little brat who was so privileged. To accompany my modest provisions on my return to school—a cutlet, the drumstick of a chicken, or one of those hard cheeses that are matured beneath wood-cinders and which one breaks into splinters with a blow from one's fist like a pane of glass—I had Chateau-Larose, Chateau-Lafite, Chambertin, and Corton which had escaped the Prussians in 1870. Certain of the wines had perished and were pale and smelt faintly of dead roses; they rested in a bed of tannin which dyed the bottles deeply; but most of them kept their fine fire, strength, and vigor. What delightful times those were! I drained the cream of the paternal cellar, glass by glass, delicately . . . My mother recorked the open bottles and contemplated the glory of the French vintages on my coloring cheeks.

How lucky are the children who do not distend their stomachs with great drafts of artificially reddened wine at meals! How well advised are the parents who dole out to their offspring an inch of pure wine—meaning "pure" in the highest sense of the word—and teach them that: "When it is not mealtime, you have the pump, the tap, the springs, and filters. Water is for thirst! Wine is, according to its quality and its flavor, a necessary tonic, a luxury, or a tribute paid to food."

Is it not also a nourishment? What lovely times those were when the natives of my village in Lower Burgundy would gather around a bottle clad in dust and cobwebs and kiss their fingers in the air to it, exclaiming—even before tasting it—"Nectar!" Do you not admit, then, that in telling you about wine here I am speaking about what I know? It is not a little thing to have learnt contempt, at an early age, both for those who drink no wine and those who drink too much.

The Vineyard and Wine are great mysteries. Alone in the vegetable kingdom, the vine gives us a true understanding of the savor of the earth. And how faithfully it is translated! It partakes of, and reveals, all the secrets of the soil. Through it we realize that even flint can be living, yielding, nourishing. Even the unemotional chalk weeps in wine, golden tears. If you transplant a vine to a distant country, it struggles to retain its personality and sometimes triumphs over powerful mineral chemicals. Gathered near Algiers, the white wines remember perfectly, for many years, the noble Bordeaux scion which sweetened them just sufficiently, softened them, and gave them gaiety. It is Madeira that colors and warms the heavy dry wine which ripens at Chateau-Chalon, on the ridge of a narrow rocky plateau.

From the grapes flourishing on the twisted vine-plant, heavy, of a transparent dull agate color, or blue and powdered with silver, the eye falls to the bare wood, like a wooden snake, wedged in between two boulders; with what, then, does this southern land feed itself, where there is no rain and which is only kept together by a network of roots? The dews of the night and the sunshine of the day are enough for it—the fire of a star, the life-sweat of another star—marvels.

What single cloudless day, what soft late rainfall decide that a vintage shall be great among the others? Human care can do almost nothing towards it: it is all celestial wizardry, the orbits of planets, sunspots.

Follow with your finger, my fair readers, on the map, beneath the eye of Nectar, the honors-list of the "years." Learn your vintage chronology and the litanies of Saints Estephe, Julien, Emilion . . . Fashion would have it so. If—still in the name of Fashion—you do not eat enough, at any rate you have lately learnt how to drink. You lack discernment and preference, and in this these charts will help you. It is sweet, merely by uttering the names of our provinces and our towns to sing the praises of the venerated vineyards. It is profitable both to the mind and to the body—believe me—to taste wine in its home, in the country which gave it all it possesses. What surprises has not a carefully thought out pilgrimage in store for you! Young wine, tried in the dim light of the wine-cellar—virgin Angevin wine, uncorked beneath a dusty bower beside a high road on a stormy summer afternoon—or exciting odds and ends discovered in an old cellar which either does not know its wealth or has forgotten it . . . From such a cellar, in Franche-Comte, I once fled as though I had robbed a museum . . . Some crazy furniture, sold by auction in a little village square included, between the dressing table, an iron bedstead, and some empty bottles, six full bottles; it was there that I made, whilst yet a young girl, the acquaintance of a Prince, fiery, imperious, and treacherous, as are all great seducers: Jurançon. These six bottles made me more interested in their country of origin than any professor could have done. I admit that at such a price geography lessons are not at everyone's beck and call. And we drank this glorious wine, one day, in the low-ceilinged parlor of an inn, so dark that we never even knew the color of the wine. Its memory is like that which a lady traveler retains of a nocturnal adventure, of the Unknown whose face she does not see, and who reveals himself only in his kisses.

Gastronomic snobbishness has given rise to a collection of Inns, such as never used to be seen. It reverences wine. Will wisdom be reborn of an unenlightened faith, confessed by mouths armor-plated by a hundred cocktails, poisonous aperitifs, withering spirits? Let us hope so. With the dawn of old age, I can offer, for my small part, the example of a stomach that has no remorse or damage, a friendly liver, and a sensitive plate, preserved by honest wine. Fill, then, Nectar, this glass which I hold out to you. A fine and simple wine as you yourself love it, you who know, giving a light bubble in which play the ruddy fires of a great Burgundian ancestor, the topaz of Yquem, the balas ruby, sometimes tinged with mauve, or violet-perfumed Bordeaux . . .

And may your slim chef of a bronzed cellarer understand me when I clink your dainty glass against a thick-sided goblet; you know well—there comes a time in life when one worships youth—that on a southern shore there is being kept for me a chaplet of wickered demijohns. One vintage fills them, the next finds them empty and fills them in its turn. Do not disdain, you who lay down fine bottles, these short-lived wines; they are clear, dry, varied, they flow evenly from the throat to the paunch and do not tarry on their way. So long as the temperament of the wine be warm, we do not care, down there, if the day be sultry, but drink great drafts of wine which refreshes us and leaves behind it a double taste of muscat and of cedarwood.

From *Prisons et Paradis,* reprinted from *Eating and Drinking: An Anthology for Epicures,* Peter Hunt, ed., 1961. London: Rainbird McLean.

England too had its Bright Young Things in the Jazz decade, but the English needed no Prohibition to make their '20s roar. Waugh, until his conversion to Catholicism sent him in search of writing "serious" literature, did for them what Fitzgerald did for the States' version.

Vile Bodies

Evelyn Waugh

Two nights later Adam and Nina took Ginger to the party in the captive dirigible. It was not a really good evening. The long drive in Ginger's car to the degraded suburb where the airship was moored chilled and depressed them, dissipating the gaiety which had flickered rather spasmodically over Ginger's dinner.

The airship seemed to fill the whole field, tethered a few feet from the ground by innumerable cables over which they stumbled painfully on the way to the steps. These had been covered by a socially minded caterer with a strip of red carpet.

Inside the saloons were narrow and hot, communicating to each other by spiral staircases and metal alleys. There were protrusions at every corner, and Miss Runcible had made herself a mass of bruises in the first half hour. There was a band and a bar and all the same faces. It was the first time that a party was given in an airship.

Adam went aloft to a kind of terrace. Acres of inflated silk blotted out the sky, stirring just perceptibly in the breeze. The lights of other cars arriving lit up the uneven grass. A few louts had collected round the gates to jeer. There were two people making love to each other near him on the terrace, reclining on cushions. There was also a young woman he did not know, holding one of the stays and breathing heavily; evidently she felt unwell. One of the lovers lit a cigar and Adam observed that they were Mary Mouse and the Maharajah of Pukkapore.

Presently Nina joined him. "It seems such a waste," she said, thinking of Mary and the Maharajah, "that two very rich people like that should fall in love with each other."

"Nina," said Adam, "let's get married soon, don't you think?"

"Yes, it's a bore not being married."

The young woman who felt ill passed by them, walking shakily, to try and find her coat and her young man to take her home.

". . . I don't know if it sounds absurd," said Adam, "but I do feel that a marriage ought to go on—for quite a long time, I mean. D'you feel that too, at all?"

"Yes, it's one of the things about a marriage!"

"I'm glad you feel that. I didn't quite know if you did. Otherwise it's all rather bogus, isn't it?"

"I think you ought to go and see papa again," said Nina. "It's never any good writing. Go and tell him that you've got a job and are terribly rich and that we're going to be married before Christmas!"

"All right. I'll do that."

". . . D'you remember last month we arranged for you to go and see him the first time? . . . just like this . . . it was at Archie Schwert's party . . ."

"Oh, Nina, what a lot of parties."

(. . . Masked parties, Savage parties, Victorian parties, Greek parties, Wild West parties, Russian parties, Circus parties, parties where one had to dress as somebody else, almost naked parties in St. John's Wood, parties in flats and studios and houses and ships and hotels and night clubs, in windmills and swimming baths, tea parties at school where one ate muffins and meringues and tinned crab, parties at Oxford where one drank brown sherry and smoked Turkish cigarettes, dull dances in London and comic dances in Scotland and disgusting dances in Paris—all that succession and repetition of massed humanity . . . Those vile bodies . . .)

He leant his forehead, to cool it, on Nina's arm and kissed her in the hollow of her forearm.

"I know, darling," she said and put her hand on his hair.

Ginger came strutting jauntily by, his hands clasped under his coat-tails.

"Hullo, you two," he said. "Pretty good show this, what!"

"Are you enjoying yourself, Ginger?"

"Rather. I say, I've met an awful good chap called Miles. Regular topper. You know, pally. That's what I like about a really decent party—you meet such topping fellows. I mean some chaps it takes absolutely years to know, but a chap like Miles I feel is a pal straight away."

Presently cars began to drive away again. Miss Runcible said that she had heard of a divine night club near Leicester Square somewhere where you could get a drink at any hour of the night. It was called the St. Christopher's Social Club.

So they all went there in Ginger's car.

On the way Ginger said, "That cove Miles, you know, he's awfully queer . . ."

St. Christopher's Social Club took some time to find.

It was a little door at the side of a shop, and the man who opened it held his foot against it and peeped round.

They paid ten shillings each and signed false names in the visitors' book. Then they went downstairs to a very hot room full of cigarette smoke; there were unsteady tables with bamboo legs round the walls and there were some people in shirt sleeves dancing on a shiny linoleum floor.

There was a woman in a yellow beaded frock playing a piano and another in red playing the fiddle.

They ordered some whisky. The waiter said he was sorry, but he couldn't oblige, not that night he couldn't. The police had just rung up to say that they were going to make a raid any minute. If they liked they could have some nice kippers.

Miss Runcible said that kippers were not very drunk-making and that the whole club seemed bogus to her.

Ginger said well anyway they had better have some kippers now they were there. Then he asked Nina to dance and she said no. Then he asked Miss Runcible and she said no, too.

Then they ate kippers.

Presently one of the men in shirt sleeves (who had clearly had a lot to drink before the St. Christopher Social Club knew about the police) came up to their table and said to Adam:—

"You don't know me. I'm Gilmour. I don't want to start a row in front of ladies, but when I see a howling cad I like to tell him so."

Adam said, "Why do you spit when you talk?"

Gilmour said, "That is a very unfortunate physical disability, and it shows what a howling cad you are that you mention it."

Then Ginger said, "Same to you, old boy, with nobs on."

Then Gilmour said, "Hullo, Ginger, old scout."

And Ginger said, "Why, it's Bill. You mustn't mind Bill. Awfully stout chap. Met him on the boat."

Gilmour said, "Any pal of Ginger's is a pal of mine."

So Adam and Gilmour shook hands.

Gilmour said, "This is a pretty low joint, anyhow. You chaps come round to my place and have a drink."

So they went to Gilmour's place.

Gilmour's place was a bed-sitting-room in Ryder Street.

So they sat on the bed in Gilmour's place and drank whisky while Gilmour was sick next door.

And Ginger said, "There's nowhere like London really you know."

Vile Bodies by Evelyn Waugh, ©1930 by Evelyn Waugh, ©1958 by Evelyn Waugh (renewed). New York: Little, Brown and Company, pp. 168–174.

*No one could make a cocktail sound as delicious as Thorne Smith, nor drunkenness as much fun. Representing all that Prohibition had tried to put a lid on, Smith's humor, by turns bawdy and sentimental, made the early Depression a lot easier for a lot of people. And gave Leo G. Carroll pre–*Man From U.N.C.L.E. *employment with the 1950s' series based on Smith's best known novel,* Topper. *Of course, the movie version gave Cary Grant a job as well.*

Rain in the Doorway

Thorne Smith

CHAPTER 7: "ESTABLISHING A LINE OF CREDIT"

By the time the last quartet of cocktails had been drained from what Mr. Owen had at first feared was going to be an inexhaustible shaker but which now he regretted was not, the partners felt themselves suitably set up to call on Mr. Hadly, the president of the bank with which the store did business in its casual way.

"We'll establish a line of credit for you, Mr. Owen," growled the Major like a jovial thunderstorm, "or I'll tear the hinges off the safe with my own two hands."

"And I'll help you," vowed Mr. Dinner. "What good is a bank unless you can establish a line of credit with it, I'd like to know?" As no one seemed prepared to tell him, he added, disgustedly, "They're so drunk I can't even hear them."

"I do feel so good," exclaimed Mr. Larkin. "I believe the four of us could establish a line of anything if we set our minds on it. What say you, Mr. Owen?"

"I say stick to credit," said Mr. Owen wisely. "Once we have our credit we can set about establishing other things—a reign of terror, for example. Some sadistic strain in my composition has always craved for a reign of terror. Also, I've always wanted to carry a can."

"Let's all carry sticks," cried Mr. Larkin. "Heavy ones. They might intimidate that skinflint, Hadly."

He rang a bell on a flower-heaped desk, a girl entered, received the order together with various flattering but uncalled-for observations from all the partners, and in a surprisingly short time returned with four heavy sticks, so large and heavy, in fact, that Mr. Dinner experienced some difficulty in handling his and himself at the same time.

"Speaking of sadism," remarked Mr. Larkin easily, slipping on a pair of light yellow gloves, "did you ever beat a defenseless child?"

In spite of the cocktails, Mr. Owen shuddered as he vigorously shook his head.

"Neither did I," went on Mr. Larkin, "but I've heard it's lots of fun."

"You might try it on my nephew," volunteered the Major. "He's an exceedingly snotty child. Last time I played cards with his father the young scamp pulled four aces from my sleeve."

"Any child should be beaten who does a thing like that," observed Mr. Dinner. "Maybe his father put him up to it."

"Quite possibly," replied the Major. "There always was a mean streak in my brother. Anyway, he'd been losing heavily all evening, what with one thing and another."

"If you'll give me a little room," put in Mr. Larkin, "I'll make an honest effort to veer myself through that door. We really must be going."

The senior partner thereupon veered through a private door giving to the street. Behind him veered his three companions, diligently swinging their sticks. Mr. Owen could not remember ever having veered onto so pleasant a thoroughfare. He drew a sharp breath and tried to remember all the things he had ever heard about Paris. This street, he felt sure, was far better than anything Paris had to offer. Surely there had never been such inviting-looking women seated at such convivial-looking tables. And as he walked past them he became inwardly elated on discovering that the women gazed at him with eyes of undisguised approval.

It was jolly to be looked at that way for a change. He could not help wondering if the cocktails had not only improved his mental outlook but also his physical appearance. If they had, he decided to become a confirmed drunkard. Too few women had paid any special attention to him in the past. Only the out-of-luck souls had seemed to drift his way. Now he was coming into his birthright. He was being admired by the opposite sex. And he, in turn, was admiring. He was returning these women's glances with brightly acquisitive eyes. He was lusting after them all. The world at last was his barnyard. Why didn't everyone get undressed and start in to chase one another? He could not decide which one he would chase first. Probably he would try to run in all directions at once.

It was a friendly sort of day, with a fair blue sky overhead. Beneath it the boulevard gave the impression of running away into friendly places. Other streets branched from it. He caught glimpses of spacious parks and plazas and lovely, interesting buildings. It seemed to be the sort of city he would have built himself, had he been given a free hand. Even the theaters wore an especially attractive aspect. One announcement read: "The only piece of cloth in this show is the curtain." Another play was called Just As We Are, and Mr. Owen, looking at the photographs of the girls, decided they would be just like that in this wholly desirable metropolis. He was very favorably impressed with everything. Delighted.

Their progress was necessarily slow, owing to the wide acquaintance of the three partners with various ladies and gentlemen they encountered in the course of their walk. Even Mr. Dinner, as small as he was and as drunk as he was, appeared to be greatly in demand. At one table Mr. Owen was introduced to a lady who in his exalted state impressed him as being the most beautiful woman in the world. When he extended his hand to take hers she deftly slipped her cafe bill into his.

"Pay that and I'm yours," she said in a thrilling sort of voice.

Mr. Larkin took the bill from the amazed Mr. Owen, scrutinized it closely, then clapped his hand to his forehead.

"Do you mean for life?" he asked the woman.

She shrugged her handsome shoulders eloquently.

"Nobody wants me for life," she replied.

"They might want you," the senior partner declared gallantly, "but, my dear, only a few men could afford to feed you. Is that just this morning's bill, or have you been living here for years?"

"You know how it is," she smiled. "Just dropped in and felt thirsty. Got a bit hungry. Ordered a few things. That's all."

"The way you say it sounds cheap as dirt," Mr. Larkin said, returning her smile with interest. "If you hadn't let us see this bill we'd never have suspected you were sitting there filled to the scuppers with five quarts of champagne—of the best champagne, let me add, not to mention various other small but costly items."

"I know," protested the woman, "but I have to act this afternoon."

"What in, a free for all?" he inquired. "Or are you fortifying yourself for the entire chorus?"

"Oh, of course," retorted the woman, "if you don't care to pay it—"

"But we do," broke in Mr. Owen.

"You mean you do," the Major amended.

Mr. Larkin quickly passed the bill to Mr. Owen.

"I don't know how much money you have," he observed, "but you'd be simply mad to have as much as that."

Mr. Owen did not have as much as that. And it was such a nice day too. A man should have no end of money on such a day as this and in the presence of such a woman. He looked about him helplessly. Mr. Larkin took the bill and called for the captain.

"Charles," he said smoothly, "this is our new partner, Mr. Owen, Mr. Horace Owen—no, I mean Mr. Hector Owen. I grow confused in the presence of so much beautifully concealed champagne. Anyway, it doesn't matter. They both begin with H. Why did I call you, Charles?"

Charles, who was evidently both fond of Mr. Larkin and quite familiar with his ways, bowed and smiled quite happily.

"Has it to do, perhaps, with the presence of Madame Gloria?" he asked.

"Tremendously, it has," cried Mr. Larkin. "The very woman herself. Now Mr. Owen, our new partner, desires very much to sign her check. He will sign the store's name and his own initials, H.O. Even I can remember them. As this bill stands now, it is a worthless scrap of paper. Signed, it becomes even more so. If it doesn't bring money, we may be able to outfit your staff. Is everything understood?"

"Fully," the captain replied with another bow.

"And Mr. Owen gets the woman," went on Mr. Larkin. "Remember that, Charles. She's his until bent with age. This is a monolithic bill. It makes one crawl to think of it. Sign, Mr. Owen, sign."

Mr. Owen signed the bill, and Charles, still smiling, departed with a generous tip provided by Mr. Dinner, who seemed to be the senior partner's peripatetic desk and cash register.

"You owe the firm five dollars in cash," said Mr. Dinner, making a note, "but you might as well give it to me."

"When he gets that line of credit," Mr. Larkin told the small man. "Which reminds me, that line is yet to be got. We must spurt. We must actually tear along."

"Thank you," said Madame Gloria sweetly to Mr. Owen. "I am yours for life."

It was exceedingly indelicate, thought Mr. Owen, the way everyone kept referring to his ownership of this woman, including the woman herself.

"We'll take that up later," he explained to Madame Gloria.

While pondering upon how fast they must tear along, Mr. Larkin had fallen into a mood of deep abstraction. At Mr. Owen's words he looked up thoughtfully.

"Did you say up or off?" he inquired. "The size of that bill makes off almost obligatory." He paused and beamed upon the fair lady. "You may call your friends back now," he said. "I've detected them hiding about in places for quite some time. You've established your line of credit. We must now establish ours. The next time you give a barbecue I hope it will occur to you to stick one of our competitors, or at least wait until we've collected the insurance for some diamonds we lost this morning. Don't know which damaged us most, you or the thief."

As they hurried from the presence of this adorable woman, Mr. Owen was dismayed to see four gentlemen and three ladies converging upon her table from various places of concealment. Then all of them sat down with cries of gladness and anticipatory expressions.

"That's the way we do things here," Mr. Larkin explained. "We boggle at nothing and nothing boggles us. A nice word, boggle. I'm of the two g's."

Mr. Larkin said so many things that made any sort of answer seem hopelessly inadequate. Hector Owen was not prepared to commit himself about boggle. He had never considered the word. However, almost any word was a good word on a day like this.

A short time later, in the office of the bank president, Mr. Owen found himself being presented to a large but florid gentleman whose impressively worried expression concealed a weak but generous character. Although habitually called a skinflint by the partners, the appellation had no justification as applied to Mr. Hadly. Anyone who did not immediately respond to the amiable proposition of their inflamed imaginations was automatically classified as a skinflint or worse.

"Well, gentlemen," he began fussily when they had seated themselves in his luxuriously appointed office, "I suppose you have called to see me about those bad checks we took the liberty of informing you about in this morning's mail."

"The liberty!" exclaimed the Major aggressively. "I call it decidedly bad taste. An imposition! Checks can't stay good forever. I say—"

"One moment, Major," cut in the suave voice of the senior partner. "Save that for later. Your words might befog the issue—even sink it entirely." Here he turned to the president and literally showered him with smiles. "You'll forgive the poor dear Major," he continued. "He's such a God damn fool. You were saying in your nice, friendly way something about checks. Ah, yes, I remember. It was something about bad checks, wasn't it? Well, let's not talk about them. We would never get anywhere that way. They're like spilled milk, no good sobbing over them. Let the dead bury the dead. And another thing, we omitted the detail of opening the mail this morning. You see, we take turns, and this morning we forgot whose turn it was. So we didn't open the mail at all. There it still is. Quite unopened. Naturally, we can't go on. You can see that for yourself, my dear, good Hadly."

"Although for the life of me I can't," his dear, good Hadly replied in a weary voice, "I'll try to if you'll endeavor to bend your brilliant faculties on this."

"Did you hear that, gentlemen?" Mr. Larkin demanded proudly. "For once a bank president has spoken the truth." He addressed himself to Hadly. "If you'll overlook those checks I'll do more than bend my faculties. I'll wrap them about anything you may have to say."

"Good!" exclaimed the president. "Wrap 'em around this. Your stockholders have placed in my hands for collection all of the guaranteed coupons for dividends due them since you first took over the store. Naturally, I must do something about it."

"I should say you must," remarked Mr. Larkin, deeply moved. "You must throw those coupons right back in their double faces. Those coupons are not worth the paper they were printed on. Never were. If the truth were known, the words printed on them are not worth as much as the paper. I didn't make up the words, anyway. As I remember, Dinner did, and he was drunk at the time. Everyone should know that a drunken man's words shouldn't ever be taken seriously. If we believed what you said when you were only half drunk you'd be owing us the bank."

"As it is," replied Mr. Hadly, unable to keep a note of bitterness from creeping into his voice, "I've practically given it to you."

"Well, we've given you things, too," put in Mr. Dinner hotly. "Shirts and socks and even the drawers to your legs. And you still owe us for a mink coat you gave to that foreign—"

"One moment," Mr. Hadly interrupted, glancing uneasily at the door. "Let's save our recriminations for the barrooms. I give you boys credit—"

"How did you know?" the Major asked in surprise. "That's just what we came for. We wanted to establish a line of credit for our new partner. And here you go giving it to us before we've even asked."

"I wish the Major were dead," said Mr. Larkin, gazing dreamily into space as if seeing laid out upon it the large, dead body of his partner. "Everything would be so much simpler then. And if Dinner would only sicken and die, I might even yet be able to snatch a few moments of happiness from life. However—" He broke off with a shrug and turned to Mr. Hadly. "I didn't want it to sound so bad when the matter was first presented to you . . . It wouldn't have sounded nearly so bad the way I was going to put it—the way I am going to put it, in fact. You see—"

"I'm not going to do it, whatever it is," the president broke in desperately. "And that's flat."

"I should say it is," Mr. Larkin agreed. "So flat it's silly. Now, listen, if you please. No more temper. I don't like it. You know how I am about temper. Easy on, easy off, or whatever you say."

Mr. Larkin stopped and looked at the president as if expecting an answer. Not knowing what else to do, Mr. Hadly nodded, although he obviously hadn't the remotest idea what he was nodding about. However, he had always found things went better if he nodded occasionally when Mr. Larkin was in full cry. The nod seemed to satisfy the senior partner, for he continued in his best manner.

"You see," he said, "Mr. Owen here, as our new partner, quite naturally has at heart the best interests of the bank with which we do business. Just how we do business and what business it is we do, need not enter into this discussion. We must all remember that. For it is very important that we should not embarrass the issue with facts. As soon as we talk facts we get to calling each other nasty names which are even harder to stand than the facts themselves. Is that understood?"

From the various expressions on the faces he inspected it was almost impossible to ascertain whether it was understood or not. Nevertheless, it was not denied.

"Very well, then," he resumed. "To continue. Mr. Owen, being who and what he is, does not want to give the wrong impression of the bank to our innumerable important friends. He does not want people to think he is dealing with a stingy bank, a penny-pinching, close-fisted, blood-sucking institution such as any bank would be that refused him a line of credit. I hope I'm not boring you with these obvious little details?"

"Not at all," said the president politely. "You've merely sickened me."

"Good!" exclaimed Mr. Larkin. "That's one way of breaking down resistance. But don't start me veering. I'd hate to begin rotating like crops." He paused and cleared his throat. "Nor," he resumed, "does our Mr. Owen want it to get about among his friends and influential business connections that the president of his bank is a man of low character, with the appetite of a swine and the instincts of a torturer. He doesn't want people to say as he passes them on the street, 'There goes old Owen, poor fellow. It's a damned disgrace how that chap's bankers keep him short of cash. I wouldn't deal with bankers like that if I had to go out of business. Hadly, from what I can learn, is a big hunk of cheese.' It would hurt him to hear things like that. It would hurt us all. But most of all it would hurt the bank. Most of all it would hurt Hadly, here, the president of the bank. And we don't want to do that."

"May I ask," inquired Mr. Hadly in a weak voice, "what you do want to do?"

"Merely to establish a line of personal credit for Mr. Owen," replied Mr. Larkin, "that would enhance the prestige of the bank we honor with our account. I will not permit it to be said that we do things on a small scale."

"You have, of course, collateral to secure this credit?" Hadly inquired more for the pleasure he would derive from infuriating the partners than from any hope of security.

"Are you mad?" three voices screamed in varying degrees of rage.

"You've already got in those beastly vaults of yours," boomed the Major, "practically everything we own in the world save our women and personal attire."

"Let's beat him up with our sticks," suggested Mr. Dinner, almost in tears. "He's gone too far this time. He'll be asking us for our list of telephone numbers next."

"No," said the senior partner. "I've got something that will hurt him more than that. When my new yacht goes into commission next week we won't invite him to come along. That will break his heart. That will simply burn him up."

"How much does he want?" asked Mr. Hadly wearily.

"How much can you spend?" Mr. Larkin promptly demanded of Mr. Owen. "I mean without stinting—without giving the wrong impression?"

"I don't know," faltered Mr. Owen. "I don't need a great deal. Never had much to spend."

"He doesn't know what he's saying," Mr. Larkin said hastily to the president. "Your sordidness has deranged him. I think he should have for his personal use about fifteen hundred a month."

"Fifteen hundred!" gasped the president. "What does he intend to do—drink, gamble, and run around with women?"

"What would you want him to run around with?" the Major demanded. "Cows?"

"I don't know," muttered the president. "I don't want him to run around at all."

"No," observed Dinner scornfully. "You want him to stay home and grow old economically."

"No, I don't," retorted Hadly. "I don't mind a man having a bit of fun now and then, but with fifteen hundred dollars a man can't have anything else but fun.

Wouldn't one thousand be enough to keep the prestige of this bank? We wouldn't expect too much, you understand."

"Let's toss a coin to see whether it's a thousand or fifteen hundred," Mr. Larkin suggested.

"All right," replied the president. "A gambling chance is better than no chance at all."

For a few moments the five gentlemen waited uneasily to see who would produce the coin. They waited without result. No one produced the coin.

"Go on," said the Major at last to Mr. Hadly. "You furnish the coin, or isn't there such a thing knocking about this dump?"

"I do wish you'd prevail upon your partners," Mr. Hadly complained to Mr. Larkin, "to moderate their manner of address somewhat. After all, I'm not quite a dog, even though I am the president of a bank. They really do owe me something."

"They owe you everything," Mr. Larkin replied hastily. "As I remarked before, it would be better were they dead and buried in their graves."

"You didn't say a word about graves," said Mr. Dinner.

"No?" asked the senior partner. "Well, I don't greatly care whether they bury you or not, so long as you're dead. However, I can't expect to get everything at once. Give me that coin, Hadly, and we'll toss for this line of credit."

"It's a half a dollar," said the banker, looking closely at the coin before handing it over. "I shall expect it back."

"God," muttered the major. "You're so damned cold blooded you could freeze ice cubes in the hollow of your tongue."

"Gentlemen," cried Mr. Larkin, tossing the coin in the air, "I cry tails."

"You would," declared the Major. "How does she lie?"

"Who?" asked Mr. Larkin, forgetting to look at the coin he had deftly caught in his hand.

"The coin! The coin!" cried the Major.

"Pardon me," said the senior partner, gazing down into his hand. "I was thinking of something else. Dear, dear me, now isn't this odd. It fell tails up. Mr. Owen, you're lucky."

"So are we," declared Mr. Dinner. "We can all borrow from him."

"But first he must have a check book," said Mr. Larkin. "Hadly, that's a dear boy, send for some check books. We all want some check books. And ask the head teller to step in. He should meet our new partner."

When the teller appeared, armed with a stack of check books, he was introduced to Mr. Owen. He was a sardonic-looking person with a pair of glittering eyes and a tongue that was awed by no man, regardless of how much he was worth.

"Not at all sure whether I'm glad to meet you or not," he told Mr. Owen. "Your partners' checks are bouncing all over the bank, and now I'll have to play leap-frog with yours, I suppose. Don't you birds ever get tired of spending money? I know I am, of trying to find it for you."

"Our new partner has lots of money to spend," said Mr. Dinner proudly. "He's just established a splendid line of credit, and he owes me five dollars already."

"Write him a check," put in Larkin, "or you'll never hear the end of it."

"And while you're settling up," Mr. Hadly suggested, "you might as well let me have that half dollar back."

"I'd like to sit next to you in hell," said Mr. Larkin admiringly to the president, "but I fear you would pick my pockets even while we shivered."

"Our hands would probably become entangled," replied Hadly, smiling at last, now that the unpleasant business was over. "Glad to have met you, Mr. Owen. Bear in mind that just because you have fifteen hundred a month you don't have to spend it all."

"Certainly not," said the Major. "We don't expect him to. We have all sorts of ideas about the disposition of his funds."

"I want a check for five berries," Mr. Dinner dully declared.

"Give him his check and let's pound along," put in Mr. Larkin. "That damned Kiarian luncheon has to be outfaced. Come along, gentlemen. We must thud. Drop round to see our new partner, Hadly, old crow. You'll find him immersed in a book in the Pornographic Department."

And with this merry leave-taking Mr. Larkin hustled his partners from the presence of the president of the most powerful bank in the city. At the door Major Britt-Britt paused and looked back at Mr. Hadly.

"When people come to see us," he announced, "especially old and valued friends, we'd consider ourselves lepers if we didn't give them a drink."

The door closed on the president's unprintable retort.

"Oh, dear me, yes," Mr. Larkin murmured happily as they strolled down the street. "That's how we do things here. It gives me a deal of pleasure to do old Hadly in the eye. Just the same, I don't believe all bank presidents are conceived in cold storage. Hadly really is a charming fellow."

"How long does this credit last?" asked Mr. Owen.

"Indefinitely, my dear fellow. Indefinitely," the senior partner assured him. "Forget all about it. We can do anything with that bank except dynamite the vaults. They wouldn't like that."

"Let's catch a spray of drinks before we join the Godly," Mr. Dinner suggested.

"Not a bad idea," said the Major.

"A good idea," agreed Larkin. "Then we'll feel better equipped to establish a reign of terror among the Kiarians."

CHAPTER 8:"THE BURNING BEARD"

"There's no doubt about it, I do feel giddy," said Mr. Larkin, giggling behind his hands as the partners pushed their way through the crush of smartly dressed gentlemen in the get-together-room of the Kiarian banqueting quarters. "At any moment now I may begin to veer like a tidy little typhoon. Don't see a face I like. They're all smug and acquisitive. Look! What is Dinner doing?"

Mr. Dinner was merely doing what appeared to be the normal thing to a drunken mind. Unable to attract the attention of his friend the Major, the little fellow, stooping over, was vigorously jabbing his cane at his huge partner between the legs of a stout gentleman. This endeavor to establish contact by means of a short cut proved effective but disconcerting. The stout gentleman, looking down to see what was disturbing him, uttered a cry of frightened amazement. What incredible metamorphosis was he going through, he wondered. In his endeavor to get away from whatever the thing was, he turned sharply and thus entangled the can between the legs of another earnest Kiarian. The Major thereupon seizing the free end of the stick gave it a violent upward tug. The shrieks of the two impaled gentlemen rang through the room. Mr. Dinner, now deeply absorbed in his occupation, which had become in his addled brain a battle of wits and deftness, yanked up his end of the cane with equal determination. The noise the gentlemen made merely whetted his enthusiasm. Even at that late date the situation might have been saved had the two Kiarians not attributed their unhappy plight to the other's deliberate intent.

"Is that a nice thing to do?" one of them, demanded furiously, endeavoring to ease himself on his objectionable as well as painful perch.

"Nice," grated the other. "You've nearly ruined me, and still you keep on doing it. Do you want to get poked in the eye?"

"I don't much care where I get poked now," the other man said in a hopeless voice. "Please stop doing it."

"I'd rather have been stabbed than to have had this happen," his vis-à-vis retorted. "If you don't take that stick away I'll do something to you."

"You are doing something to me already," cried the stout man. "You're doing plenty. Don't wiggle it like that."

"But he isn't doing it at all," a Kiarian spectator helpfully informed the speaker.

"Oh, dear," Mr. Larkin observed reflectively to Hector Owen. "Dinner can think of the damnedest thing to do with a stick. Those gentlemen must be in great distress."

"I hate to think of it," said Mr. Owen. "Look how the Major's pulling. He'll cut those men in two."

From the sounds the men were making this was not difficult to believe. Drink had lent strength to Dinner's arms and added to that already possessed by the Major's. The gentlemen, turning on the stick, were imploring their tormentors to abandon this contest in which they themselves had never expressed the slightest desire to participate.

"Oh, very well," said the Major to his small partner. "You can have your old stick."

With this he abruptly released his hold, and the two gentlemen fell weakly to the floor, from which they were presently assisted by a number of sympathetic Kiarians.

"Certainly I'm going to have my stick," little Dinner declared stoutly. "And no big bully is going to take it away from me either."

"May I ask," inquired Mr. Larkin, "how you managed to get two Kiarians on the end of your stick?"

"They got themselves there," said Dinner. "I didn't get them there. Must have thought they were playing horse. I think some of these Kiarians drink too much. Come along. Let's get our badges."

Without even so much as glancing at the tortured men, Mr. Dinner led the way to a table at which an official was importantly giving out badges bearing the Christian name or the nickname and the occupation of the member presenting himself. The senior partner received a badge which informed the world he was "Larkie" and that he passed his days as a merchant. This trophy he immediately pinned on the back of an innocent bystander. Mr. Dinner's was affixed with strategic craft by the Major to the seat of another gentleman's trousers. Whenever he bent over, this gentleman announced to the gathering at large that he made a practice of referring that section of his body simply as Lu. The Major, with much unneccessary adjusting, pinned his badge on the breast of a pretty cloakroom girl who did not seem to mind. Taking it all in all, Mr. Owen decided his partners were men with excessively puerile minds and futile ways. Why they had insisted on their badges and waited in line to get them only to make them objects of ridicule and derision was more than even his somewhat confused mind could understand.

On the way to the luncheon room they were accosted by numerous members who, in spite of the absence of badges, addressed the partners in cloyingly familiar terms, anyway.

"Well, B.B.," cried one gentleman, clapping the Major on a shrinking shoulder. "It does my eyes good to see you, old boy. How's the Little Lady?"

"You must be not only dumb but also blind," the Major told him. "If you ever saw my wife you'd damn well know she wasn't little, and if you'd ever heard her line of talk you'd never call her a lady. Go fawn on somebody else. I don't like that way of talking."

As surprised as he was at the display of brutal frankness on the part of the Major, Mr. Owen was even more so by the language of Mr. Dinner. A gentleman named Buddy was addressing the small man in hearty accents.

"Hello, Lu," this person cried. "Tickled to death to see you."

"You're a liar," said Dinner coldly. "You know you hate my guts."

And with this he turned his back on the much discomfited Buddy. Another well meaning Kiarian had cornered the glowering Major.

"It isn't the heat," this man was saying, "it's the hu—"

But the man never finished his sentence. The Major knocked him down with a single blow, wiped his hand with an expensive silk handkerchief delicately scented with eau de Cologne, and deliberately walked away.

"We can't let them get too friendly with us," Mr. Larkin informed the astounded Owen. "If we did, they'd ruin our lives."

"I don't see why they want to know you at all," said Mr. Owen, "if you treat them that way."

"You don't know Kiarians," the senior partner replied. "They'd forgive a murder for the sake of prosperity and sell their wives for a boom in business."

"What do you think of our city, Mr. Owen?" a person calling himself Benny wanted to know a few minutes later, during the course of an introduction.

"Tell him it smells," whispered Mr. Dinner, at Mr. Owen's shoulder. "I want to watch his face."

"It smells," said Mr. Owen obediently, and he, too, watched Benny's face. It merely became more foolish, if possible, than it had been before he asked the question.

"You should never have brought him along," Benny told Mr. Larkin when he had recovered from the shock. "He'll never mix with the boys."

"Go away," said Mr. Larkin in a dead voice, "or I'll pull your inquisitive nose."

"But I didn't mean it smells, really," Mr. Owen explained when the man had tottered off.

"I know," replied Mr. Larkin, "but it does when he's around. If you say the first thing that comes into your head at one of these luncheons you're pretty sure to be right."

"Why do you ever come?" asked Mr. Owen.

"To annoy people," said Mr. Larkin, "and to be annoyed in turn. It's good for everybody. Yet sometimes, when I come away from one of these luncheons, I get the feeling it must all have been a dream—that these people didn't really exist but were culled up from a fit of depression. Why, they even sing at one. All together they sing—boosting songs, patriotic songs, mother songs. You'll hear them soon yourself."

Mr. Owen did, and although there was too much of it and the songs were either too optimistic or sentimental, he had to admit to himself the singing was pretty good. Nevertheless, he wished it would stop.

Mr. Larkin enlivened his table by surreptitiously pouring some essence he had purchased for his cigarette lighter into his neighbor's glass of water. The other partners were as innocent of this affair as was the owner of the water himself. And the owner was a personage of note, a man high up in the deliberations of the Kiarians. His inspirational speeches were listened to frequently and indefinitely. He was a man with a long square beard, lots of white to his eyes, and a deep, beautiful voice. He was large and he was lofty. He was the president of one of the most progressive advertising agencies in town and had grown used to having himself referred to by his initials which through some trick of fate chanced to be W. C. Just previous to the serving of the soup this magnificent gentleman felt himself called upon to discover how well his voice sounded in public today. Accordingly he rose, and with a fat hand holding an unlighted cigar, silenced the singing mouth.

"Kiarians!" he cried. "I am no longer your chairman, your leader."

"Good!" croaked a disguised voice from somewhere in the neighborhood of the sleepy-looking Mr. Dinner.

The bearded gentleman paused, frowned heavily, then filled his lungs with air.

"Kiarians!" he burst forth again, and Mr. Dinner, who had been perfecting the art in secret, promptly began to quack like a duck.

"Kiarians!" cried the man. "Is there a duck in this room?"

"You haven't begun on your soup yet," said the Major in a loud admonitory voice. "What do you want with a duck?"

"I don't want a duck," thundered W. C.

"But you did ask for a duck," said the Major, stubbornly sticking to his guns.

"I asked if there was a duck," the man retorted.

"Well, is there?" Mr. Larkin inquired pleasantly.

"How should I know?" snapped the great man. "There were duck-like sounds in the room. If it wasn't a duck I'll eat it."

"May I eat it if it is?" the Major asked brightly.

"What!" exploded the man. "I have no duck for you to eat. I want to get rid of this duck."

"Will somebody please throw that duck out," Mr. Larkin called in a voice of authority, then murmured to Mr. Owen, "Isn't this amusing? It's better than I hoped."

"What duck?" asked several earnest voices.

A volley of unpleasant sounds shattered the brooding silence of the room. Mr. Dinner, startled himself by his remarkable performance, appeared from behind his napkin and looked about him with an innocent face.

"Kiarians!" called W. C., now at the end of his patience. "You speak as if I personally knew this duck, as if deliberately I had brought this duck among you, as if this duck were my boon companion." He paused, then flung at them, "How should I know what duck?

"Lord love a duck!" cried Dinner for no apparent reason.

W. C. shivered. His temper was out of hand.

"I hate a duck," he shouted. "I'd like to wring its neck." A fresh burst of protesting quacking from Dinner greeted this impassioned avowal.

"There it goes again!" cried W. C. "Am I to be mocked by this pest of the barnyard?"

"Maybe he's in your beard," suggested major Britt-Britt in a penetrating voice, "and is squawking to get out. I know I would if I were a duck."

"I wish to God you were," thundered the incensed Kiarian, "and in the barnyard, where you belong."

"You'd be the first worm I'd gobble," said the Major with surprising self-control, and added thoughtfully, "Even if it killed me."

"Kiarians!" once more cried the bearded gentleman, who had never before been talked down by any man and who proudly refused to be defeated at the bill of a fowl. "Now that the duck has stilled its brazen voice I will again raise mine."

Mr. Dinner was quacking tearfully behind his napkin, but the great man pretended not to hear the sounds. Mr. Larkin was watching him closely, waiting for that inevitable moment when the hand would raise the glass of water to the bearded lips. That moment was not far off. The senior partner held a match pressed to the side of a match box.

"Kiarians!" thrilled the orator's voice, his hand reaching for the glass. "I no longer govern your deliberations."

The glass was raised slightly from the table. "I no longer give you the light—"

Mr. Larkin struck, and as if performing some well polished feat of legerdemain W. C. lifted a flaming glass which promptly ignited his beard. The applause in the room was tremendous. Kiarians rose and cheered. They had never before suspected good old W. C. of such ability in sleight-of-hand. Admirers in the room cried out, but none cried louder than W. C. himself.

"Don't applaud, you damn fools!" he shouted through the fumes and smoke. "Somebody put me out!"

"Do you mean throw him out?" the Major inquired lazily. "Like the duck, for instance?"

Mr. Dinner, in his drunken excitement, was quacking unrestrainedly. Mr. Owen, still undecided whether he was witnessing a trick or a burning Kiarian, remained quietly in his seat. The senior partner had risen and was holding a bowl of soup carefully poised beneath the burning beard.

"Now," he said in a voice of great composure, "if you'll be so good as to lower your head a trifle, then plunge the beard in this bowl of delicious soup, I think we'll have you extinguished in a jiffy. It would be better if you closed your eyes. The fumes will be terrific, I fear."

But before closing his eyes W. C. caught a vivid picture of the city's greatest advertising leader solemnly dipping his glorious beard into the depths of a bowl of soup. What an imperishable memory he would leave in the eyes of the assembled Kiarians! This was the end of his career as a public character. He could never hope now to complete the autobiography which one of his copy writers was doing for him on office time and without extra pay. The eyes he turned on the senior partner were filled with rage and hate.

"What do I care," he growled, "if the soup is delicious?"

Making a virtue of necessity, he bared his teeth in the semblance of a smile for the consumption of the watching Kiarians, then plunged his beard in the soup. Even as he did so, thoughts of moving-picutre comedies of the slapstick variety flashed through his mind. There was a sizzling sound and a burst of smoke and through it all gleamed the white teeth of the advertising genius whose lips were contorted in a maniacal grin. Strong men caught their breath, while weak ones turned away. Mr. Dinner quacked like a duck and sleepily rubbed his eyes. One especially enthusiastic Kiarian cheered in a loud voice, a well meaning display which only seemed to increase the mental anguish of the smoldering man.

"The beard is now extinguished," Mr. Larkin announced. "Pardon me if I cry a little. W. C.'s personally conducted bonfire has made my eyes water."

"It's fairly sickened me," commented the Major in a rough, coarse voice. "Barring none, that beard is the worst I've ever smelled. I'll bet it hasn't been dusted off since Queen Victoria died."

This observation on his personal habits of cleanliness was too much for W. C. He raised his massive head and glared at the Major. The beard emerged from the delicious soup tastefully garnished with vegetables and spaghetti. Mr. Owen, for the sake of his own sensibilities, was moved to offer the gentleman a napkin.

"You wouldn't look quite so awful," he said in a sympathetic voice, "if you used this on what's left of those whiskers."

Automatically W. C. accepted the napkin and thoughtfully applied it to his damaged beard.

"May I do it for you?" Mr. Larkin asked, advancing on the man. "I'd dearly love to dry your poor dear beard."

The advertising genius started back with a cry of horror. The sparks of madness were gleaming in his eyes.

"I'll dry my own beard," he cried through wisps of smoke still straining through the hard dying tangle of hair. "Keep your hands off it. Don't come a step nearer."

"You wouldn't have to ask me twice," Major Britt-Britt informed the world. "It certainly is a mess."

"About the most revolting beard I ever saw," claimed little Mr. Dinner. "I wish he'd hide it somewhere."

"And I wish the lot of you would stop saying things about my beard," the great man retorted. "It's bad enough to have it burned, without having it discussed."

"That's right," agreed Mr. Larkin. "No beard looks its best immediately after a fire. We expect too much of W. C. He's done enough as it is."

At this point Mr. Mark Crawly, universally known as Big Boy, presiding officer of the local Kiarians, deemed it expedient to introduce some semblance of order into all this acrimonious chaos. Mr. Crawly was a nice chap. One could not help liking him a little. He possessed what all Kiarians loved most—a fine front. Inside, Mr. Mark Crawly was just plain dumb, which was no handicap among his fellow members. He could say stupid things in a firm, manly voice and get away with them. Years ago his firm had recognized the value of his smile as a business getter and had elevated him to the position of general sales manager. It occasionally took new members of his staff almost a month to discover that he had only a vague idea of what it was all about. He smiled business in and competition down. Above his desk was a Keep Smiling sign. In the Nut and Bolt Trade Journal his words were often quoted. " 'Meet depression with a grin and smile a boom into being,' says Mark Crawly at the Tenth Nut and Bolt Convention." Had it not been for his hard-working subordinates he would have smiled his firm into bankruptcy, but that, of course, was not generally known. Big Boy Crawly now addressed the still slightly smoldering W. C. in particular and the room in general.

"Gentlemen," he began, "we all like and respect our W. C."

Mr. Dinner giggled a little at this, but Mr. Crawly frowned.

"We are sorry about his beard," he resumed, "yet even now I'm not sure whether he did it on purpose or not."

An animal-like howl burst from the advertising man's singed lips.

"Do you think I'd deliberately set fire to my beard," he asked in an impassioned voice, "to amuse you damn fools?"

"I assumed you were trying to amuse us," Big Boy Crawly replied good-naturedly. "It was funny, you know. How did it catch?"

"It was very dry," announced Dinner in a solemn voice. "That beard was a public menace."

"It was nothing of the sort," shouted W. C. "I've worn that beard for years."

"When was it last dry cleaned?" Major Barney inquired.

"It never was dry cleaned," retorted the other.

"I feared as much," said the Major. "The damn thing burned of its own accord like a heath fire. Spontaneous combustion sort of—that's how I figure it out."

"The Major means," Mr. Larkin explained to the room, "that the regrettable fire which broke out in the beard was due to the accumulation of years of debris. Am I right, Major?"

"As always," the big chap replied. "Wonder if he had it insured?"

"Was the beard insured, W. C.?" the senior partner inquired, turning politely to that infuriated gentleman. "Not against theft, of course, but for fire?"

"Bah!" ejaculated W. C. "Bah!"

"He's bleating like a sheep," cried Mr. Dinner, who was professionally interested in animal noises. "There's no end to the things the man can do."

"One moment," called Mr. Crawly. "I asked W. C. a simple question, and you gentlemen have made the thing seem terribly involved. W. C., can you tell us how your beard caught fire?"

"How should I know?" shot back the mighty man in the agony of his soul.

"Aren't you even interested?" Major Barney asked innocently. "I know if I had a beard and it happened to go off like yours did, I'd never rest until I'd discovered the cause. The damn thing might do it again."

"It would be awful to have it happen in bed with a woman," Mr. Dinner observed reflectively. "What would she think?"

W. C. sprang to his feet. Beard or no beard, he would put a stop to this. These people were not going to continue talking about himself and his beard as if neither of them were present.

"Kiarians!" he cried, showing the whites of his eyes. "Let's abandon this talk about beards and turn to other things."

"We haven't settled that matter of the duck yet," Mr. Dinner suggested. "We might take that up."

"Someone was making duck noises," W. C. replied. "I've thought that out, too. There is no duck."

The volley of quacking and squawking that greeted this denial far surpassed all previous demonstrations. W. C. paused and shook himself like a punch-drunk fighter.

"I may as well sit down," he observed at last in a hopeless voice, "if that duck is going to interrupt every word I say."

"It seems to be coming from the direction of your table," a Kiarian called out.

"You look under the table, Dinner," the major commanded, "and I'll look under whatever remains of his beard. That duck must be one place or the other."

"If you touch my beard I'll cut your throat!" cried W. C., grabbing up a knife.

"A pretty way for a man to talk," complained Mr. Dinner. "We were only trying to help."

"I wasn't going to touch his old beard," explained Major Barney in an injured voice. "I was just going to peep under it."

"Kiarians!" almost screamed the distracted man. "Are you going to allow these ruffians to turn this dignified meeting into a discussion of my beard? Are you going to permit them to torture me about it—to throw my beard in my face?"

"Better than burning it in ours," put in Major Barney.

"Very well, then," called out the senior partner in a conciliatory voice. "Let's table the beard now that he's finished souping it."

"How do you do that?" asked the unintelligent Dinner. "Do you mean flatten it out and iron it?"

"Bah!" exclaimed the great leader. "And bah again."

"Why again?" asked Major Barney. "We heard the first bah, and it didn't mean anything either. I like the duck better."

.Mr. Dinner lifted his napkin and behind it quacked his thanks. W. C., with a despairing cry, flung up his hands and sank heavily to his chair. Then he brought his hands down and rested his head in them. He would never appear in public again, he vowed to himself. But he did. He appeared many times until at last he died in public and had a public Kiarian funeral and then was promptly and publicly forgotten as such men should be.

He could never have been tolerated in private.

 This is a place for family and friends, and to drink and be happy together.
—MICHELLE DOWNIE, WAITRESS, LONGFELLOW'S WAYSIDE INN, WAYSIDE INN ROAD, SUDBURY, MASSACHUSETTS

From *The Thorne Smith 3-Decker* by Thorne Smith, © 1948. Garden City, NJ: Doubleday Sun Dial edition, pp. 510–535.

Like Machen, H. P. Lovecraft is best known as a horror writer. Unlike him, he was a teetotaler. But this grave handicap did not prevent H.P.L. from penning the following verse, which perfectly evokes the eighteenth-century drinking song.

Drinking Song from "The Tomb"

H. P. Lovecraft

Come hither, my lads, with your tankards of ale,
And drink to the present before it shall fail;
Pile each on your platter a mountain of beef,
For 'tis eating and drinking that brings us relief:
    So fill up your glass,
    For life will soon pass;
When you're dead ye'll ne'er drink to your king or your lass!

Anacreon had a red nose, so they say;
But what's a red nose if ye're happy and gay?
Gad split me! I'd rather be red whilst I'm here,
Than white as a lily—and dead half a year!
    So Betty, my miss,
    Come give us a kiss;
In hell there's no innkeeper's daughter like this!

Young Harry, propp'd up just as straight as he's able,
Will soon lose his wig and slip under the table;
But fill up your goblets and pass 'em around—
Better under the table than under the ground!
    So revel and chaff
    As ye thirstily quaff:
Under six feet of dirt 'tis less easy to laugh!

The fiend strike me blue! I'm scarce able to walk,
And damn me if I can stand upright or talk!

Here, landlord, bid Betty to summon a chair;
I'll try home for a while, for my wife is not there!
So lend me a hand;
I'm not able to stand,
But I'm gay whilst I linger on top of the land!

From *Fungi from Yuggoth and Other Poems* by H. P. Lovecraft. © 1963 by August Derleth. Renewed 1971. New York: Ballantine Books, pp. 52–53.

The first woman in this anthology, Craig Rice was a brilliant mystery writer; but both her heroes and villains were, as a rule, heavy drinkers. She herself knew of what she wrote. Her work deserves to be much better known, and it is a pleasure to feature it here.

8 Faces At 3

Craig Rice

"I want to go to the Casino and hear Dick's band," Helene said.

"In those blue pajamas?" said Jake indignantly. "Hell's bells, woman, don't you own any other clothes?"

They had found Malone sleeping peacefully in Jake's room, wakened him by holding an opened bottle of rye under his nose. Now they were draped about the room—Jake comfortably settled in the one easy chair, Malone sprawled on the bed, and Helene lying flat on the floor. It had, she said, a reassuringly immobile quality which the furniture lacked. It wheeled a little, but it did not spin.

"I won other clothes," she said, "but nothing as fetching as these pajamas. Still if you don't like them, I can always take them off."

"You two fools are drunk," Malone said hastily.

" 'Malone says Dick's deb not guilty,' " Jake read from the pile of afternoon papers heaped on the floor, and made a mental note to keep the last editions away from Dick and Malone. He picked up another. " 'Band Leader's Bride Didn't Murder Aunt, Lawyer Says.' "

"Well, is she guilty?" asked Helene from the floor.

"Of what?"

"Auntycide."

"What do you think?"

"Hell, no."

"Personally," Jake said, "I think Helene did it and she's just trying to confuse us."

"Do you confuse easily?" Helene asked in a dangerously dulcet tone.

Malone rose to his feet a little unsteadily. "I have things I ought to be doing."

"Sit down," Jake snapped. "Don't leave me alone with her."

Malone sat down heavily.

"It seems to me," he said a little severely, "that you two are taking this pretty damned lightly."

"I always take these things lightly," Helene told him. "I'm not the romantic type."

"I'm talking about the murder."

"Just a single-track mind," Jake said, digging under the pile of newspapers for the bottle. "It's over, isn't it? The old lady's dead and we can't bring her back. Personally I wouldn't if I could."

"I want to go to the Casino and hear Dick's band," Helene repeated.

"In the pajamas?"

"In them or out of them. Let's toss a coin, like the young man did to decide whether to visit a phrenologist or go to see his girl."

"What have you got on under them?" Malone asked in a disinterested tone.

"You're not on a witness stand," Jake reminded her. "Don't let him intimidate you."

"I don't intimidate worth a damn." She managed to get on her feet. "But watch this." She pulled the pajama legs loose from her garters so that they fell gracefully about her ankles, wrapped her coat about her person and stood artfully posed like a debutante about to be photographed at the opening night of the opera. "Do I have on an evening gown?"

"You have," said Jake. "By God, you have."

"These pajamas have been everywhere," she told him convincingly.

She began intensive operations with facial cream, powder, an eyebrow brush, and a deadly looking lipstick. They watched until she folded the contents of a small-sized beauty parlor into her handbag. "Tell me, John Joseph, did Holly do it or didn't she?"

"No," said Jake Justus.

"You're a hopeless minority," Malone said.

"You damned fool," Jake said indignantly. "You heard her story."

"She was alone in the house with the old lady," Malone began slowly and a bit thickly. "Her brother and the Parkinses are gone. She hated her aunt. Had hated her for years, was afraid of her. The old woman had terrified her, had deliberately terrified this fragile, delicately reared girl. Now she approaches a crisis in her life. Something snaps in her brain and—"

"Save it for the jury," Jake reminded him.

"Shut up. Anyone looking at what happened last night, seeing it lucidly and coldly and calmly, can see it was the product of a disordered mind. The clocks. The telephone call. Making Glen's bed and Parkins' bed. Some deep psychological significance in that. Going up and stabbing the old woman three times. Why three? Opening the window. Why? And then fainting away at the old woman's feet. That's where they found her."

"You forget," said Jake, "who made her bed. She was in it when she woke up. Who—"

"She *says* she was in it."

"Damn you, Malone. We'll get another lawyer. Who made her bed? Some roving chambermaid on the loose, I suppose. Or she slept on the floor. No, Malone, it won't wash."

"I want," said Helene stubbornly, "to go to the Casino and hear Dick's band."

Dick Dayton, at the Blue Casino, led his band with an unthinking, mechanical precision. The music seemed to come from very far away, through a mist, the figures on the dance floor were so many wound-up dolls. In the intermissions, he was vaguely conscious of people talking with him, but the words they said could not penetrate the fog that encircled him.

Jake had told him to see it through. Swell publicity, Jake said. Those people out on the dance floor knew what had happened—they knew that his girl, his bride, was held for murder in the Blake County jail. They knew it and they sympathized, and they saw him here in front of his band trying to act as though nothing had happened and not succeeding very well, and it was swell publicity, Jake said. The hell with Jake. He didn't have the faintest idea what the boys were playing.

Why had she done it? Or had she done it? If he only knew. If he could only talk with her again, if she would only tell him the truth. But they wouldn't let him talk with her alone. God! Would he ever be alone with her again? If they convicted her, would they allow her an hour alone with him before they led her down the corridor to the electric chair? *Christ!*

The baton snapped in his hand. Steve came up, offered to take over, he waved him away.

This was to have been their first night together. Now he was here and Holly was in a cell in the Blake County jail. Holly in a cell. Holly in a cell, perhaps for life. And he going to see her on visiting days. Perhaps after twenty years or so they would pardon her. Half a lifetime off for good behavior. Well, he'd be waiting for her—forever if he had to.

Could Malone get her out of this? Jake seemed to think so. Jake was a smart guy. Malone seemed to think so, too. The trial would be swell publicity, wonderful publicity, marvelous publicity. God, what publicity! Damn Jake Justus. Sure they'd acquit her. Malone knew his stuff. Not guilty by reason of temporary insanity. An acquittal on the first ballot. Hell, yes!

And then would she tell him the truth? Would she tell him if she'd gone up to that room and taken the little knife in her hand and crept up to the helpless old woman and thrust that knife into the withered old bosom, again and again and again?

Would he ever know?

Ah! There was Jake. Jake, and John J. Malone, and that gorgeous, beautiful, magnificent blonde wench. Not in the same class with Holly, no. But terrific. Where the hell had they all been? She looked like a queen in the evening wrap, with just enough of her blue evening gown showing. Blue evening gown hell! Those pajamas!

He began to laugh, too loudly.

Steve stepped up, took the baton from his unresisting hand, and gently shoved him in the direction of Jake's table. Dick nodded gracefully.

Easy, he kept telling himself, easy. Don't let them know, don't let them see. He pretended they were a table of important customers, smiled, bowed, and sat down with them.

"Well, how goes it?" He managed to say it casually, hoping they wouldn't have any news, no news that he couldn't bear hearing.

"Going! It's gone! We know she didn't do it. Malone isn't even going to let it come to trial." Dick didn't see the warning glance Jake gave Malone.

"Sure," Helene said, kicking Jake under the table, "she's practically out of jail right now!"

"Drink, Dick?"

"No, thanks. I'm not drinking."

"You'd better," said Malone thickly, "you'd better have one with us, to celebrate."

"Hell, yes," Jake added, "you've got to celebrate. She didn't do it. The rest is mere formality."

"—parts Benedictine, two parts Metaxa brandy, and a dash of orange bitters,"

Helene was saying to the waiter. She smiled briskly at Dick. "I ordered that for you, babe."

"What is it?"

"A little invention of my own. I call it the Chicago Fire."

There was no doubt she had named it correctly.

"Jake, you meant it?" Dick asked after the third Chicago fire. "She didn't do it? You're telling me the truth?"

"You don't think I'd lie to you about a thing like this!"

Helene interrupted with a question about the orchestra. Then Jake began telling stories; John J. Malone began telling stories. Then a black-haired wench in a bright yellow dress came from somewhere and attached herself to them, especially to John J. Malone. Everything began to get a little dim.

Somehow they all got out of the Casino and into a taxi. How it was achieved, not even Jake knew. There was Brown's where Helene won six-eighty-five in a slot machine and spent it on drinks for the house; Lucky Joe's where the wench in the yellow dress and Helene insulted each other; the Blue Door where Jake lost seven-fifty at dice with the bartender; the Rose Bowl where John J. Malone got into a fight with a stranger from Rock Island.

Dick was not quite sure what was going on. It should have been a swell evening, a hell of a swell evening. But every time he began to feel at little at home in his surroundings, there was that terrible, aching remembrance of Holly in jail, Holly, his girl. And tonight, of all nights since the beginning of time!

At those times Helene would put a glass in his hand and he would drink it, Jake would remind him that they were celebrating, and John J. Malone would mumble, "Sure, we'll have her out of there tomorrow."

They went to Johnny Leyden's, where John Joseph Malone got into a fight with a perfect stranger from South Bend and lost the collar off his shirt; to the 885 Club where Dick managed to get Holly off his mind long enough to substitute hilariously at the piano; to Riccardo's, where Helene sang in a surprisingly good voice to the tinkling guitar; to a black and tan on the south side. Somewhere along the way they lost John J. Malone—they never did find out where.

By that time Dick was aware, now and then, that something was terribly wrong with his world, but it was difficult to remember what it was. Something that had to do with some girl.

They went cruising madly along the drive in a taxi, and he remembered it all suddenly and terribly, and knew that they had been lying to him all along, and there was something he wanted to tell Jake, because Jake was his friend. Then everything became very dim indeed and the interior of the taxi became a deep dark well in which he was being drowned, and he felt Jake's hand reaching out to catch him as he fell.

"We certainly took care of that situation in a hurry," said Helene, looking down at Dick. They had driven back to the hotel where, with the help of a bellhop and a taxi driver, Dick had been tucked into his bed.

Helene looked at him for a long moment.

Rumpled and pink-faced, his eyelids swollen, he looked like a small boy who had cried himself to sleep.

"He doesn't know anything about it," Helene murmured. "He'll remember, when he wakes up in the morning. He'll wake up knowing that something is wrong, but he won't know what it is, and then little by little he'll remember until it all comes back to him, all of it."

Suddenly she bent over the bed and kissed him lightly on the forehead.

Then they went across the hall, to Jake's room. Jake found two drinks hidden in a bottle tucked away under his clean socks. The room was silent, deathly silent. There had been much noise, much excitement, much disturbance. Now it was very late, and incredibly quiet.

Jake looked at the girl. What did one do under the circumstances? A Miss Brand of Maple Park was a bit outside his ken. This sharp edge of the moment stuff was always bad. What were her views on the subject anyway?

"Tell me," he said, stumblingly, and again, "tell me."

For just one moment she was sober, cold sober. Something crossed her face that hurt, that even hurt him, looking at her. He saw the same terror in her eyes that he had seen in Nellie Parkins' eyes.

"What is it?" he said sharply. *"What do you know?"*

"Don't ask that! Don't ask that again!"

"I won't." He meant it.

He looked at her closely. Her face was frozen, her eyes had a curiously jellied look.

"My God," he said to the empty air, "you're out as cold as a clam." He caught her as she fell.

He carried her across the room, deposited her on the bed, wondered what to do about, or with, the blue pajamas, decided to leave them where they were, covered her with a blanket, and began thinking about what Holly Inglehart Dayton had done or hadn't done the night before.

Sometime later he struggled out of a half doze, looked at the blonde head on his pillow, wondered whose it was and how it had gotten there, glanced at his watch. It was three o'clock.

He sat bolt upright. She opened half an eye.

"Now I remember what it was I wanted to know!"

She muttered a remark that was either highly pertinent or highly impertinent, or both. He didn't hear it.

"What stopped the clocks?"

And then, peaceably and without another word, he passed silently out.

John P. Marquand chronicled the decline of the WASP upper classes in such serious books as The Late George Apley. *In* Life at Happy Knoll, *he dealt with that class's doing at a Country Club. In this chapter, he shows that, no matter how incompetent, a bartender may keep the keys to far more than the liquor cabinet.*

Should Auld Acquaintance Be Forgot?

John P. Marquand

A letter from Mr. Roger Horlick of the Board of Governors of the Happy Knoll Country Club to Mr. Albert Magill, President Emeritus, regarding the maintaining of the status quo of the men's bar and continuing the employment of its present barkeeper.

DEAR ALBERT:

As you know, there has been agitation recently, chiefly among the younger and less well-established members of the Happy Knoll Country Club whose names appear only too frequently on the bulletin board for nonpayment of house bills, to get Old Ned out of the men's bar at Happy Knoll and to renovate the whole place. The idea is, in accordance with the argot of a generation younger than ours, that the men's bar—where your father and mine used to have their toddies after a hard afternoon on the links—stinks.

Indeed, in a sense the men's bar does, in that almost two generations of excellent hard liquor have spilled upon its woodwork, creating an aroma which binds the past to the present. The word among several of our more successful young executives, however, is that the men's bar is archaic. They want the mirrors, the beer steins and the canvas of "The Frightened Nymph" by Bouguereau to be removed, and the bar and the brass rail and the two brass cuspidors along with them. In their place, they suggest something more like a Paris bistro or sidewalk cafe with high bar stools, artificial awnings and artificial sunlight. The clique that is most vociferous in demanding this change is headed by a young advertising man named Bob Lawton, whose election to the Board of Governors at Happy Knoll still remains to me a mystery. Granted that every element of our somewhat varied membership should, ideally, be represented, one must stop somewhere.

I don't know how well you know young Mr. Lawton, but probably very well if you have ever met him, because he is constantly thrusting out his hand and saying, "The name is Bob Lawton and it's time we got to know each other better." At any rate, it is the idea of our Bob Lawton to "live it up a little in the bar." Primarily he proposes to have a sign over its door called "Fun 'n' Games Room for Men Only," and a scale of chromatic neon lighting which will change at various hours and a number of gambling machines arranged in what he calls a "comedy manner," the proceeds of which will go toward refurbishing the bar, which is now run at a deficit. Without consulting anyone, he has already, during a recent trip to Paris, collected some humorous French drawings of a scatological nature as wall decorations. The only one that I can now recall depicts a frightened dachshund looking at a wet umbrella which is distributing a puddle on the floor. "Mon Dieu," the dog is saying in French, "they will think it is I."

But the thing that really upsets me is the move afoot to get rid of poor Old Ned, who, as barman, is the spirit of the place itself. It is said correctly that Ned, in spite of his almost forty years of loyal service at Happy Knoll, would never have been made head barkeeper here if Henri Racine had not been stolen under our very noses by the Hard Hollow Country Club. Old Ned is willing to tell anyone that he came to Happy Knoll as a local boy who did odd jobs on the golf course under Old Angus. He was admittedly never good with anything mechanical. Even today he often strips the gears of the electric mixer when he attempts to make a daiquiri. It is also true that Ned only became a barboy after he sprinkled salt on the 18th green, mistaking it for fertilizer. It is true that when Henri was abstracted in a most unsportsmanlike manner, Ned could not mix drinks as well as Henri. Indeed as of today if you ask for a Scotch Ned is only too apt to give you rye, and he pours quinine water into highballs instead of soda. His eyesight is not what it used to be and his coordination, never good, has not recently improved. Annually he gets more flustered at Saturday night dances and he is more and more prone to leave the bar and let younger members take his place.

But none of this is really the point. The point to consider is the loyalty, the friendship and deep interest that Ned has always shown for every member of Happy

Knoll for whom he has ever mixed a beverage, including that member's private life and his most confidential business affairs. Through the years Ned has developed an intuitive skill in estimating the incomes and inclinations of our members, and he is a walking encyclopedia about their pasts. Good Old Ned! I do not mean for a moment that he talks out of school. Up to date he is the most closemouthed individual in existence and under the proper circumstances will, I am sure, remain so. He has been and always must be a permanent feature of Happy Knoll. I frankly would not care to envisage my future or that of many others with Old Ned employed somewhere else, say in the bar or dining room at Hard Hollow.

You may think that I am implying that Old Ned is prying and inquisitive. I do not intend such a nonfactual criticism for a single moment. But he does radiate an atmosphere of unalloyed human sympathy, which Dr. Fosbroke, our psychiatrist member, only the other day said he wished that he might emulate. Old Ned has only to nod his kind bald head, surrounded now by his austerely close-clipped white hair, to elicit immediate confidence. I am aware of this myself. Indeed I am often surprised, later, on recalling things I have told Old Ned about Mrs. Horlick and our married daughter and our son's recent disastrous marriage. I have wondered sometimes whatever had induced me, not that I am worried for a moment about his discretion. He has never asked me a single question. Nevertheless, Old Ned plus even one Old-fashioned is often equal to an hour on the couch of a Vienna-trained analyst. The men's bar would not be the same place at all without Old Ned. It would cease to be a sanctum of the soul.

It is, of course, a truism that alcohol is apt to unleash loquacity, but there is more than this in the redolent atmosphere of the men's bar at Happy Knoll when, after a day on the links, or even the card room, Old Ned, behind that genial length of mahogany, offers you a glass. For one thing, you never can be sure how much will be in it. Sometimes I do suspect that the dear old rascal deliberately plays favorites and plies those who interest him most with more Happy Knoll spirits than he does the others. After all, can anyone—even you or I—enjoy everyone equally? And after all, must there not be long, dull periods in any bar like Happy Knoll where business, save for week ends and holidays, is seldom brisk until late afternoon? For instance, Old Ned, it would seem, has recently developed a great fondness for Mr. Bert Byles, a new member of ours from Foxrun Road, and I can hardly blame Old Ned for this partiality after his hours of polishing and breaking glasses in a completely silent room, with all his friendly instincts frustrated. Mr. Byles, it seems, is an unusually outgiving person with an active thirst for sympathy, and he is beset by extreme difficulties, both personal and financial. It always does a lot of good to speak your troubles and to have Old Ned nod silently, and I may say in passing that other men's bar patrons are interested in the troubles of Mr. Byles, too, because he suffers out loud more eloquently than anyone else. Besides, it is very hard, I have found, in any barroom anywhere, to avoid becoming deeply interested in another's domestic difficulties, since these always fall into the patterns that are in the nature of a common experience. But under the grave attention of Old Ned such disturbed confessions assume a new depth and a new value not unlike the program of a radio mediation hour.

As a small example of what I mean, it seems that Mrs. Byles is addicted to what one might term pursuit by telephone. Frequently Mr. Byles has been said to retreat to the bar weeping when he is being paged in other portions of the club, but when he sees Old Ned with a bottle of bitters in his hand he knows that all is well.

Under Old Ned's auspices the men's bar at Happy Knoll is what General MacArthur might rightly term a "privileged sanctuary" for all husbands suffering from telephonic persecution. When the bar telephone rings and Old Ned answers, you know that you are safe. His voice, which in his best years was hoarse and unmusical, now carries a conviction all its own. Even a Happy Knoll wife who knows that her husband is in the bar believes momentarily that he is not, when she hears Ned speak. It may be, as frequently happens, that she will call again five minutes later, but you are still safe because of Old Ned's magic. His negative is firmer on the second call, carrying with it an undertone of outraged dignity. Few wives except Mrs. Byles ever call a third time.

It has occasionally struck me as odd that Old Ned should have great difficulty in adding up his bar checks, because he actually has a fine head for business combinations. Our fellow member H. J. Culbertson would be the first to agree with this statement. You may remember that some years ago H. J. absorbed Pasqual Power in a rather spectacular manner. The transaction, as H. J. himself confessed to me later, had placed him under a very considerable nervous strain and, in seeking relaxation, he adjourned to the bar at Happy Knoll.

Without H. J.'s ever knowing how it happened, he found himself telling of the whole transaction to Old Ned, including certain details which H. J. frankly confesses he had never even told his lawyers. He still says that he is amazed and that Old Ned might have a "half nelson" on him if Old Ned should ever wish to use it. The truth was that Old Ned understood every one of the details that H. J. told him. It is a touching tribute to him that H. J. has never worried for a single moment. The bar at Happy Knoll still is a privileged sanctuary.

It should be a source of pride to the club that an enormous amount of important business has been transacted in the bar. The stock of the P. W. Brakeweight Company moved to a new majority ownership right under Old Ned's nose, aided by a few Manhattans but mostly by Old Ned's benign exterior. Several of our best tax lawyers have advised their clients regarding some very interesting methods of business deduction in the bar. There is no doubt that the membership of Happy Knoll comprises one of the finest groups in the world, but even at Happy Knoll there are mysteries. There is a family whose name I won't mention living on Foxglove Lane that broke up almost overnight. Old Ned knows the reason. A certain home on Willowrun Path burned very suddenly two years ago. Old Ned can tell you whether or not this fire was entirely accidental. You have undoubtedly heard repercussions of a fist fight in the card room last winter. Old Ned could tell you the reasons and the details, blow by blow—if he could be induced to talk. But as someone said there, only the other day—after choking down a third of Old Ned's whisky sours that were mixed for some reason with ginger ale—nothing ever gets by Old Ned but nothing ever gets through him either.

I must assure you quite frankly, Albert, that I am not retailing hearsay gossip. I know these things about Old Ned because he told them to me yesterday and a good deal more besides. It seems that poor Old Ned is just as worried as you and I are by this new element that wants to do over the men's bar. Poor Old Ned, who does hear everything, has of course heard that a small clique wants a newer, defter barkeeper. Naturally this makes him deeply disturbed, I might even say upset, and never in the years I have known him have I heard him talk as freely as he has in the last few days. In fact, he put his own case very eloquently to me only the other evening.

"I am close friends with many lovely and very important members at Happy Knoll," he said. "I think if you was to speak to them about me, they would hate to see me leave."

Frankly, I echo those sentiments, and I am willing to bet a lot of the old crowd and even some of the new crowd will, too. Happy Knoll would not be the same place without Old Ned. His disappearance would give a lot of members, including myself, a very real attack of mental anguish. I do not mean that Old Ned would not be a true-blue Happy Knoller no matter where he might end up, but I know you will agree with me he had better stay right here. It is true that he is not improving. It might be well to have a younger man to mix the drinks, but let's keep Old Ned behind the bar.

Several of us are already circulating a petition to this effect, and you may be interested to know that Mr. H. J. Culbertson, Mr. Byles, five of our best corporation lawyers and one of our bank presidents have not only signed but are calling up their friends. In fact, the sentiment for keeping Old Ned is becoming a landslide. The subject will be discussed at the next meeting of the Board of Governors. I don't think there will be any difficulty, but it might be as well if you would write a confirming letter, since you have been around the bar a good deal yourself. All you need to say is: "Should auld acquaintance be forgot? Keep Old Ned."

Cordially yours,

ROGER HORLICK

 Make the Martinis dry, the whiskey "Bushmill's," and your drinking partner, ME!
—MARK FELICETTI, SENIOR MANAGER, THE MAGIC CASTLE 7001 FRANKLIN STREET, HOLLYWOOD, CALIFORNIA

From *Life at Happy Knoll* by John P. Marquand, 1955, 1956, 1957. New York: Little, Brown, & Company, pp. 55–67.

Lucius Beebe was, like Marquand, a chronicler of WASPish decline. Unlike J. P., however, he had no intention of going gently into that good night. These pieces appeared in the San Francisco Chronicle, *from which publication Beebe waged ceaseless war against liberals, teetotalers, and bad taste of all descriptions.*

A Drinker's Observations

Lucius Beebe

THE WISDOM OF POLONIUS

In May 1922, I first took passage to cross the Atlantic in the Cunard steamship *Aquitania,* then at the apex of its celebrity as a luxury vessel of the type spoken of in the public prints as "an ocean greyhound." As a youth traveling alone, I was assigned, as was the custom of the time at capacity sailings, to share a stateroom with another gentleman whose identity was revealed as that of Claude Graham-White.

At this remove the name may mean little except to students of aviation, but Graham-White was a flying pioneer of impressive dimensions, so valued by the English government as an expert and consultant that he was paid an annual sum, reported to be $25,000, never to set foot in an airplane. He was a handsome, sophisticated and urbane *viveur* in whose debt I shall always stand for many kindly offices of worldliness.

Learning, conversationally, that I was an undergraduate at New Haven and that this was my first trip abroad, my roommate was quietly amused and remarked: "I think you will learn more that will be useful to you in life in six days aboard a Cunard steamship than in a semester at any university in the world."

Claude Graham-White couldn't have been more right. Others may sit at the feet of Yale or Oxford or the Sorbonne as their alma mater, but although I am a graduate elsewhere and have latinate documents to attest to it, I own to being a graduate first and foremost of transatlantic travel and the University of Cunard.

A good deal of gin has flowed under the bridgework since Claude Graham-White instructed me in some of the basic facts of life: gentlemen wear shawl collar dinner jackets, peaked lapels are for musicians (this was 1922); only show-offs drink more than one bottle of champagne at breakfast; the most costly cognac on the wine list isn't always the best; don't ask for Maine lobster on an east-west passage or English channel sole going from west to east; tip the carver at Simpson's no more than threepence.

Don't get in fist fights with Frenchmen, which is insulting, strike them with your walking stick; try not to use the words "bottom" or "bum" in polite English society; they mean something else. When the King of Spain asks you to have a drink in the Ritz Bar, which he will probably do if you're a regular, it's more polite not to order a King's Death, which is what he himself will be drinking, but to call it a Royal Highball.

Nearly 40 years afterward these instructions may, to some, seem vaguely frivolous. In 1922 they were the wisdom of Polonius.

THE EXPATRIATE DRINKER

That sterling repository of our national yesterdays, American Heritage, has just released an issue devoted in its literate and pictorial entirety to the 1920s, in all probability the last era in the record that is available to being viewed as a well defined and clearly identifiable entity.

I find no mention of one of the great manifestations of the time which should be at least a footnote to any history of prohibition and its attendant infamies.

I speak, of course, of the expatriate drinker.

As clearly defined and as articulate in his grievance against the Yankee homeland as any literary or esthetic rebel who found spiritual consolation and fulfillment on the Left Bank, the alcoholic exile was a part-time refugee from the American wasteland who has not received his historic due in the annals of the period.

His spiritual home was the Ritz Bar on the Cambon side of that auspicious Paris hostelry. His money was, to be sure, unassailably in dollars and he might either be a commuter aboard the then weekly sailings of the Olympic, Berengaria or Paris or he might establish semi-permanent residence in France. Often enough he was explicitly patriotic in every aspect of national temperament excepting for what came in bottles. There he was red revolutionary, tracing his ancestry to the participants in the Boston Tea Party and the great Whiskey Rebellion in Pennsylvania. He was often homesick, eagerly questioning the latest arrivals from the Atlantic sea lanes and shuddering at the gruesome details of life and death in the speakeasies of the homeland.

Among the platinum-plated expatriates of the Ritz Bar there grew up a body of legend and folklore while their ritualistic drinking was surrounded with protocol. It was a men's bar exclusively at noontime and women, among them Connie Bennett and Marion Davies, were, much against their inclination, herded by the management into a smoke-filled female groggery across the corridor variously known as the Dog Kennel and the Black Hole of Calcutta.

The thirsty but mannered regulars assembled outside the entrance to the Ritz Bar as noontime approached awaiting, as it were, the noonday gun to start the day's serious drinking. To be seen inside the place before noon identified you as a certifiable alcoholic and no-gooder. To be late was unfashionable, with the result that when Count Johnny Perdicaris looked at his wrist watch and shouted "Now" a small man could be maimed in the ensuing crush.

Strict protocol was observed in seating the devotees of the men's bar itself. Banquettes on the left as one entered were reserved for young gentlemen from Yale, Harvard, Princeton and the members of the American Embassy staff presided over by Myron Herrick. Those to the right were occupied exclusively by South Americans, stiffly starched, pomaded and tightly buttoned, a long row of heavy-rimmed single eyeglasses, mostly with poodles.

Many of the Ritz Bar regulars like Donald Rogers, a former member of the consular service, had been trapped there for years. Rogers was notorious for engaging passage on each successive boat and then not making it until the clerks at Cunard and White Star no longer made actual reservations for him.

Red letter days at the Ritz Bar were those when Alfonso, regnant King of Spain, and his friend Berry Wall, king of the dudes, came in for a drink known in His Majesty's absence as a King's Death but called a Royal Highball when he was present. It comprised a quart of ice cold champagne in a large glass with a generous slug of vintage cognac and a handful of fresh strawberries for panache. His Majesty allowed this was a refreshing beverage with which to begin the day and wiped his mustaches on a king-sized handkerchief from Charvet's just across the way with a crown in the corner. Your correspondent admired these and one day the King gave him one which is still in the bank vault in Reno.

It may do as an index of the time. Our heroes were still kings and there were kings around to be heroes.

A SLUR ON AMERICAN MANHOOD

About the only one of Dr. Genevieve Kupfer's findings on alcoholism which will raise any eyebrows, blood pressure or Martini glasses is the unequivocal definition by the lady doc of a heavy drinker as anyone who drinks three times a week and takes three or more belts of Old Reprehensible at a time. The inextinguishable mirth this lady-like appraisal would have aroused in the circles of my youth, a period when the American people, 160 million strong, stayed drunk as sailors for thirteen long years in the Second American Revolution called prohibition, would have been deafening.

I know, I know, the heroic exploits of other times grow in the telling and assume a dimension that tends to magnify the original fact. Sordid love scuffles in dreary roadhouses assume the perfumed overtones of the Lunts in "Reunion in Vienna."

Shore dinners at Connecticut beach resorts, with a gallon of warm gin under the table and a bathroom handy for the universal emesis that accompanied its consumption gleam through the mists of antiquity like Trimalchio's Feast. Or at least like supper with Henry VIII and Cardinal Wolsey having at whole roasted steers and tossing pheasant carcasses under the table while regiments of pages did a double scurry with sack and Rhenish to appease the royal thirst.

Still and all, Dr. Kupfer's three drinks at a time were widely consumed between breakfast and luncheon by undergraduates of my acquaintance at Cambridge and New Haven, and the universal highball was so deplored by the university authorities that the reading rooms at Baker Memorial Library at Harvard were equipped with abruptly sloping book-rests to discourage whiskey as an accompaniment to economics.

Bradley Fisk and Bydie Kilgour, who lived in lordly affluence in Apthorp House, filled a three gallon water cooler with fresh gin every morning and kept open house so that friends on the way to Music 1 (The History of Roman Band Instruments) or noble Professor Kitteredge's course in Shakespeare might arrive in a state elevated to that of the theme of their instruction.

The Beacon Street hostess or patroness of a debutante ball at the Somerset who estimated the capacity of her guests at three belts of the ardent or less than a bottle each of the product of the Champagne never entertained a second time.

But not even the magnifying glass of time can conceivably paint the lily of alcoholic heroism that found its finest hours in the Fakirs' Ball annually staged by Cynthia White or the Harvard-Yale boat races in June which could easily have been rowed in the spilled drinks which swirled ankle-deep on the ballroom floor at the Griswold Hotel in New London.

When, inevitably, at three in the morning, the police backed the wagon up to Webster Hall to remove Miss White's revelry, in toto, to jail, extra patrol wagons had to be borrowed from as far away as the Bronx. At New London, with the passage of years, the yacht basin in front of the Griswold became marked on navigational charts as of unsound anchorage because it was floored with a parquet of empty bottles.

These were the glory years of rebellious patriotism and American manhood when the three drinks of Dr. Kupfer's modest assessment were consumed by a large devoted segment of the population as the merest eye-opener or phlegm-cutter in preparation for a hard day's work at the barricades, which were of solid polished mahogany. The happy insurrectionists were generaled by as splendid a staff as ever directed a war effort, all named Tony, Mike, Eddie and Lou and whose insignia of rank was a white apron and bar rag. The definition of hard drinking in those heroic times only included the patriot who, every day of his life, was carried from the field of battle, inanimate on a shutter before noon.

LET'S HAVE A RUM-SOAKED BALLOT

One of the most preposterous impositions that has come to be established by entrenched and vindictive bigotry at the expense of milquetoast American taxpayers and voters is the pestilential practice of making it impossible to get a drink in public on election day. Through the agency of this vicious harassment, and since it includes primaries and by-elections, a couple of days out of every year in most States are irrevocably chalked up as triumphs for meddlesome bureaucrats and the insensate snouters of prohibition.

The basic fear behind this pigsty assertion of bigotry is, according to its apologists, that the unwary voter treading a sober and reflective measure toward the polling place might be accosted by solicitous villainy bent on defiling the purity of his franchise and swerving him from emplacing the mark of his choice on the ballot.

In other words, his vote might be purchased for a noggin of squareface.

If votes can be bought for liquor and a price in proof bourbon be set on the ballot, then the ballot is being elevated beyond any status it now owns.

No other limit or hindrance is placed on the influencing and outright purchase of the voter's suffrage with promises of pie in the sky and limitless freedom to pillage his betters through the swindles of social legislation. Political campaigns in the United States are nothing but a universal scheme for the corruption of registered voters with promises which, happily, no politician has the slightest intention of fulfilling.

He can be promised the distribution of cash bonuses from the treasury for his vote, he can be promised the right to tax his neighbor into bankruptcy, to ruin the credit of the Nation, or he can be promised free false teeth and the universal medication of his ailments from paresis to hemorrhoids for his vote, but he may not be solicited with a Martini or shot of bourbon and branch.

Advocates of civic responsibility are loud in powerful exhortations to get out the vote but take no note of the melancholy fact that no man's judgment is as keen or his purpose as pure as when he has taken a belt or two at the nearest bar before getting into a scuffle with the ballot.

This is the heart of the matter. Nothing scares the living daylights out of a politician like the idea of an intelligent appraisal of his candidacy by the electorate. A realistic appraisal induced by alcohol might well reveal him for the fraud and potential thief he is. Hence no booze. Keep the voter sober and stupid at all costs.

As long as American elections were floated on the sea of hard liquor our sanctimonious snouters now profess to find so shocking, fair winds filled the sails of the Ship of State and all prospects for the future were golden. At an all-time low in the ebb of our national destinies, when the future is no more than a day-to-day gamble, we might well revert to the conduct and institutions of our forefathers, at least for a day. There's nothing in the world to lose.

OTHER TIMES, OTHER MORIARITYS

Because he is evidently and amply aware of the uses of publicity and sees to it that no accredited reporter ever gets a check even if he's been bathing in Bollinger, an amiable saloonkeeper in New York named P. J. Moriarity is by way of becoming a national character.

But to an older generation of serious drinkers, Moriarity's doesn't mean P. J.'s no doubt agreeable sluicing premises.

It meant the address at 216 East Fifty-eighth street where Dan Moriarity and his brother Mort ran New York's most celebrated and certainly most respectable masculine speakeasy throughout most of the Twenties and until repeal of the infamy that made them rich, respected and, by many loyal customers, beloved.

Dan and Mort were old time East-Side New York Irish. They spoke with a brogue, had important connections in the right police and political circles and drank their own whiskey. Their customers were the elite of New York's masculine saloon set, professional advertising and newspapermen, well-mannered cut-ups and the less impulsive and more solvent undergraduates of New Haven and Princeton who lived within commuting distance and spent the evening there as educationally as in the university library.

Dan tolerated neither breaches of the peace nor of gentlemanly rectitude. You held your liquor or you didn't come back. At 216 there was the conventional steel-sheathed door under a brownstone stoop with Judas hole, chains and throw bolts and the customers could be cased in the light of a glaring arc lamp which providentially was in just the right location in the all-brownstone block. Or maybe Dan had it put there.

A daily regular at four every afternoon was Charlie McCrae who came up from Wall Street on the East Side subway and refused to speak to anyone, even his own brother at the bar, until Mort or Dan had served him a triple Martini which he inhaled at a single swallow. After he had had three of these benevolent arrangements he went home to have cocktails with his family.

There were two prices at Dan's: two bits for the O'Gradys, Currans and other neighborhood Irish, and six bits for Vanderbilts, Mellons and Whitneys of whom there were many and thirsty, too. Martin Curran, the doorman at a nearby apartment house, was the only non-Catholic Irishman Dan admitted and on one occasion Martin, slightly in wine, shattered the usually well-bred tranquility of the place by booming: "Dan, could a Protestant bastard buy one for the house?"

Another doorman regular was Joe O'Grady, who called carriages at Bendel's and whose uniform was so magnificent that he was once introduced by Sherman Hoyt to some visiting British yachtsmen as "Admiral O'Grady of the U.S. Navy" without arousing suspicion.

Sunday mornings Dan's was Manhattan's leading temple of the hangover, the sufferers crouching motionless and noiseless at the bar, many of them with silk top hats resting on the hatrack by the door preparatory to passing the plate at St. Thomas's or St. Patrick's, trying to get up courage to take the first sip of brandy milk punch that would make or destroy them. It was forbidden to drop a pin lest the noise shatter the therapeutic silence.

When closing hour came at night, usually about three o'clock, Dan or Mort or whoever was on varied the honored British call of "Time, gentlemen" with the query, "Have you no homes?" Many of us had no homes but Dan's and I wish I could hear him say it again.

From *The Provocative Pen of Lucius Beebe, Esq.*, 1966. San Francisco: Chronicle Publishing, pp. 7–8, 48–50, 67–68, 90–92.

Ray Bradbury is, to put it simply, one of our greatest living national authors. But while such works as The Martian Chronicles *and* Something Wicked This Way Comes *have established him in the public mind as a Science Fiction and Fantasy writer, this selection shows another side to him—gentle evoker of nostalgia.*

Dandelion Wine

Ray Bradbury

The town, later in the day.

And yet another harvest.

Grandfather stood on the wide front porch like a captain surveying the vast un-motioned calms of a season dead ahead. He questioned the wind and the untouchable sky and the lawn on which stood Douglas and Tom to question only him.

"Grandpa, are they ready? Now?"

Grandfather pinched his chin. "Five hundred, a thousand, two thousand easy. Yes, yes, a good supply. Pick 'em all. A dime for every sack delivered to the press!"

"Hey!"

The boys bent, smiling. They picked the golden flowers. The flowers that flooded the world, dripped off lawns onto brick streets, tapped softly at crystal cellar windows and agitated themselves so that on all sides lay the dazzle and glitter of molten sun.

"Every year," said Grandfather. "They run amuck; I let them. Pride of lions in the yard. Stare, and they burn a hole in your retina. A common flower, a weed that no one sees, yes. But for us, a noble thing, the dandelion."

So, plucked carefully, in sacks, the dandelions were carried below. The cellar dark glowed with their arrival. The wine press stood open, cold. A rush of flowers warmed it. The press, replaced, its screw rotated, twirled by Grandfather, squeezed gently on the crop.

"There . . . so . . ."

The golden tide, the essence of this fine fair month ran, then gushed from the spout below, to be crocked, skimmed of ferment, and bottled in clean ketchup shakers, then ranked in sparkling rows in cellar gloom.

"Dandelion wine."

The words were summer on the tongue. The wine was summer caught and stoppered. And now that Douglas knew, he really knew he was alive, and moved turning through the world to touch and see it all, it was only right and proper that some of his new knowledge, some of this special vintage day would be sealed away for opening on a January day with snow falling fast and the sun unseen for weeks or months and perhaps some of the miracle by then forgotten and in need of renewal. Since this was going to be a summer of unguessed wonders, he wanted it all salvaged and labeled so that any time he wished, he might tiptoe down in this dank twilight and reach up his fingertips.

And there, row upon row, with the soft gleam of flowers opened at morning, with the light of this June sun glowing through a faint skin of dust, would stand the dandelion wine. Peer through it at the wintry day—the snow melted to grass, the trees were reinhabited with bird, leaf, and blossoms like a continent of butterflies breathing on the wind. And peering through, color sky from iron to blue.

Hold summer in your hand, pour summer in a glass, a tiny glass of course, the smallest tingling sip for children; change the season in your veins by raising glass to lip and tilting summer in.

"Ready, now, the rain barrel!"

Nothing else in the world would do but the pure waters which had been summoned from the lakes far away and the sweet fields of grassy dew on early morning, lifted to the open sky, carried in laundered clusters nine hundred miles, brushed with wind, electrified with high voltage, and condensed upon cool air. This water, falling, raining, gathered yet more of the heavens in its crystals. Taking something of the east wind and the west wind and the north wind and the south, the water made rain and the rain, within this hour of rituals, would be well on its way to wine.

Douglas ran with the dipper. He plunged it deep in the rain barrel. "Here we go!"

The water was silk in the cup; clear, faintly blue silk. It softened the lip and the throat and the heart, if drunk. This water must be carried in dipper and bucket to the cellar, there to be leavened in freshets, in mountain streams, upon the dandelion harvest.

Even Grandma, when snow was whirling fast, dizzying the world, blinding windows, stealing breath from gasping mouths, even Grandma, one day in February, would vanish to the cellar.

Above, in the vast house, there would be coughings, sneezings, wheezings, and groan, childish fevers, throats raw as butcher's meat, noses like bottled cherries, the stealthy microbe everywhere.

Then, rising from the cellar like a June goddess, Grandma would come, something hidden but obvious under her knitted shawl. This, carried to every miserable room upstairs-and-down would be dispensed with aroma and clarity into neat glasses, to be swigged neatly. The medicines of another time, the balm of sun and idle August afternoons, the faintly heard sounds of ice wagons passing on brick avenues, the rush of silver skyrockets and the fountaining of lawn mowers moving through ant countries, all these, all these in a glass.

Yes, even Grandma, drawn to the cellar of winter for a June adventure, might stand alone and quietly, in secret conclave with her own soul and spirit, as did Grandfather and Father and Uncle Bert, or some of the boarders, communing with a last touch of a calendar long departed, with the picnics and the warm rains and the smell of fields of wheat and new popcorn and bending hay. Even Grandma, repeating and repeating the fine and golden words, even as they were said now in this moment when the flowers were dropped into the press, as they would be repeated every winter for all the white winters in time. Saying them over and over on the lips, like a smile, like a sudden patch of sunlight in the dark.

Dandelion wine. Dandelion wine. Dandelion wine.

 I walked Criswell [famed TV psychic of the 1950s and 60s] home a few times—
even when he couldn't walk!
—BARTENDER, BOARDNER'S, 1652 NORTH CHEROKEE, HOLLYWOOD, CALIFORNIA

Dandelion Wine, © 1975 by Ray Bradbury (most recent . . .), revised Bantam Edition, published by arrangement with Doubleday in January, 1976, pp. 12–15.

The Guy with the Eyes

Spider Robinson

Callahan's Place was pretty lively that night. Talk fought Budweiser for mouth space all over the joint, and the beer nuts supply was critical. But this guy managed to keep himself in a corner without being noticed for nearly an hour. I only spotted him myself a few minutes before all the action started, and I make a point of studying everybody at Callahan's Place.

First thing, I saw those eyes. You get used to some haunted eyes in Callahan's—the newcomers have 'em—but these reminded me of a guy I knew once in Topeka, who got four people with an antique revolver before they cut him down.

I hoped like hell he'd visit the fireplace before he left.

If you've never been to Callahan's Place, God's pity on you. Seek it in the wilds of Suffolk County, but look not for neon. A simple, hand-lettered sign illuminated by a single floodlight, and a heavy oaken door split in the center (by the head of one Big Beef McCaffrey in 1947) and poorly repaired.

Inside, several heresies.

First, the light is about as bright as you keep your living room. Callahan maintains that people who like to drink in caves are unstable.

Second, there's a flat rate. Every drink in the house is half a buck, with the option. The option operates as follows:

You place a one-dollar bill on the bar. If all you have on you is a fin, you trot across the street to the all-night deli, get change, come back and put a one-dollar bill on the bar. (Callahan maintains that nobody in his right mind would counterfeit one-dollar bills; most of us figure he just likes to rub fistfuls of them across his face after closing.)

You are served your poison-of-choice. You inhale this, and confront the option. You may, as you leave, pick up two quarters from the always-full cigarbox at the end of the bar and exit into the night. Or you may, upon finishing your drink, stride up to the chalk line in the middle of the room, announce a toast (this is mandatory) and hurl your glass into the huge, old fashioned fireplace which takes up most of the back wall. You then depart without visiting the cigar box. Or, pony up another buck and exercise your option again.

Callahan seldom has to replenish the cigarbox. He orders glasses in such quantities that they cost him next to nothing, and he sweeps out the fireplace himself every morning.

Another heresy: no one watches you with accusing eyes to make sure you take no more quarters than you have coming to you. If Callahan ever happens to catch someone cheating him, he personally ejects them forever. Sometimes he doesn't open the door first. The last time he had to eject someone was in 1947, a gentleman named Big Beef McCaffrey.

Not too surprisingly, it's a damned interesting place to be. It's the kind of place you hear about only if you need to—and if you are very lucky. Because if a patron, having proposed his toast and smithereened his glass, feels like talking about the nature of his troubles, he receives the instant, undivided attention of everyone in the room. (That's why the toast is obligatory. Many a man with a hurt locked inside finds in the act of naming his hurt for the toast that he wants very much to talk about it. Callahan is one smart hombre.) On the other hand, even the most tantalizingly cryptic toast will bring no prying inquiries if the guy displays no desire to uncork. Anyone attempting to flout this custom is promptly blackjacked by Fast Eddie the piano player and dumped in the alley.

But somehow many do feel like spilling it in a place like Callahan's; and you can get a deeper insight into human nature in a week there than in ten years anywhere else I know. You can also quite likely find solace for most any kind of trouble, from Callahan himself if no one else. It's a rare hurt that can stand under the advice, help and sympathy generated by upwards of thirty people that care. Callahan loses a lot of his regulars. After they've been coming around long enough, they find they don't need to drink any more.

It's that kind of bar.

I don't want you to get a picture of Callahan's Place as an agonized, Alcoholics Anonymous type of group-encounter session, with Callahan as some sort of salty psychoanalyst-father-figure in the foreground. Hell, many's the toast provokes roars of laughter, or a shouted chorus of agreement, or a unanimous blitz of glasses from all over the room when the night is particularly spirited. Callahan is tolerant of rannygazoo's; he maintains that a bar should be "merry," so long as no bones are broken unintentionally. I mind the time he helped Spud Flynn set fire to a seat cushion to settle a bet on which way the draft was coming. Callahan exudes, at all times, a kind of monolithic calm; and U.S. 40 is shorter than his temper.

This night I'm telling you about, for instance, was nothing if not merry. When I pulled in around ten o'clock, there was an unholy shambles of a square dance going on in the middle of the floor. I laid a dollar on the bar, collected a glass of Tullamore Dew and a hello-grin from Callahan, and settled back in a tall chair—Callahan abhors barstools—to observe the goings-on. That's what I mean about Callahan's Place: most bars, men only dance if there're ladies around. Of one sex or another.

I picked some familiar faces out of the maelstrom of madmen weaving and lurching over honest-to-God sawdust, and waved a few greetings. There was Tom Flannery, who at that time had eight months to live, and knew it; he laughed a lot at Callahan's Place. There was Slippery Joe Master, who had two wives, and Marty Matthias, who didn't gamble any more, and Noah Gonzalez, who worked on Suffolk County's bomb squad. Calling for the square dance while performing a creditable Irish jig was Doc Webster, fat and jovial as the day he pumped the pills out of my stomach and ordered me to Callahan's. See, I used to have a wife and daughter before I decided to install my own brakes. I saved thirty dollars, easy . . .

The Doc left the square-dancers to their fate—their creative individuality making a caller superfluous—and drifted over like a pink zeppelin to say Hello. His stethoscope hung unnoticed from his ears, framing a smile like a sunlamp. The end of the 'scope was in his drink.

"Howdy, Doc. Always wondered how you kept that damned thing so cold," I greeted him.

He blinked like an owl with the staggers and looked down at the gently bubbling pickup beneath two fingers of scotch. Emitting a bellow of laughter at about force eight, he removed the gleaming thing and shook it experimentally.

"My secret's out, Jake. Keep it under your hat, will you?" he boomed.

"Maybe you better keep it under yours," I suggested. He appeared to consider this idea for a time, while I speculated on one of life's greatest paradoxes: Sam Webster, M.D. The Doc is good for a couple of quarts of Peter Dawson a night, three or four nights a week. But you won't find a better sawbones anywhere on Earth, and those sausage fingers of his can move like a tap-dancing centipede when they have to, with nary a tremor. Ask Shorty Steinitz to tell you about the time Doc Webster took out his appendix on top of Callahan's bar . . . while Callahan calmly kept the Scotch coming.

"At least then I could hear myself think," the Doc finally replied, and several people seated within earshot groaned theatrically.

"Have a heart, Doc," one called out.

"What a re-pulse-ive idea," the Doc returned the serve.

"Well, I know when I'm beat," said the challenger, and made as if to turn away.

"Why, you young whelp, aorta poke you one," roared the Doc, and the bar exploded with laughter and cheers. Callahan picked up a beer bottle in his huge hand and pegged it across the bar at the Doc's round skull. The beer bottle, being made of foam rubber, bounced gracefully into the air and landed in the piano, where Fast Eddie sat locked in mortal combat with the "C-Jam Blues."

Fast Eddie emitted a sound like an outraged transmission and kept right on playing, though his upper register was shot. "Little beer never hoit a piano," he sang out as he reached the bridge, and went over it like he figured to burn it behind him.

All in all it looked like a cheerful night, but then I saw the Janssen kid come in and I knew there was a trouble brewing.

This Janssen kid—look, I can't knock long hair, I wore mine long when it wasn't fashionable. And I can't knock pot for the same reason. But nobody I know ever had a good thing to say for heroin. Certainly not Joe Hennessy, who did two weeks in the hospital last year after he surprised the Janssen kid scooping junk-money out of his safe at four in the morning. Old Man Janssen paid Hennessy back every dime and disowned the kid, and he'd been in and out of sight ever since. Word was he was still using the stuff, but the cops never seemed to catch him holding. They sure did try, though. I wondered what the hell he was doing in Callahan's Place.

I should know better by now. He placed a tattered bill on the bar, took the shot of bourbon which Callahan handed him silently, and walked to the chalk line. He was quivering with repressed tension, and his boots squeaked on the sawdust. The place quieted down some, and his toast—"To smack!"—rang out clear and crisp. Then he

139

downed the shot amid an expanding silence and flung his glass down so hard you could hear his shoulder crack just before the glass shattered on unyielding brick.

Having created silence, he broke it. With a sob. Even as he let it out he glared around to see what our reactions were.

Callahan's was immediate, an "Amen!" that sounded like an echo of the smashing glass. The kid made a face like he was somehow satisfied in spite of himself, and looked at the rest of us. His gaze rested on Doc Webster, and the Doc drifted over and gently began rolling up the kid's sleeves. The boy made no effort to help or hinder him. When they were both rolled to the shoulder—phosphorescent purple I think they were—he silently held out his arms, palm-up.

They were absolutely unmarked. Skinny as hell and white as a piece of paper, but unmarked. The kid was clean.

Everyone waited in silence, giving the kid their respectful attention. It was a new feeling to him, and he didn't quite know how to handle it. Finally he said, "I heard about this place," just a little too truculently.

"Then you must of needed to," Callahan told him quietly, and the kid nodded slowly.

"I hear you get some answers in, from time to time," he half-asked.

"Now and again," Callahan admitted. "Some o' the damndest questions, too. What's it like, for instance?"

"You mean smack?"

"I don't mean bourbon."

The kid's eyes got a funny, far-away look, and he almost smiled. "It's . . ." He paused, considering. "It's like . . . being dead."

"Whooee!" came a voice from across the room. "That's a powerful good feeling indeed." I looked and saw it was Chuck Samms talking, and watched to see how the kid would take it.

He thought Chuck was being sarcastic and snapped back, "Well, what the hell do you know about in anyway?" Chuck smiled. A lot of people ask him that question, in a different tone of voice.

"Me?" he said, enjoying himself hugely. "Why, I've been dead is all."

"S'truth," Callahan confirmed as the kid's jaw dropped. "Chuck there was legally dead for five minutes before the Doc got his pacemaker going again. The crumb died owing me money, and I never had the heart to dun his widow."

"Sure was a nice feeling, too," Chuck said around a yawn. "More peaceful than nap-time in a monastery. If it wasn't so pleasant I wouldn't be near so damned scared of it." There was an edge to his voice as he finished, but it disappeared as he added softly, "What the hell would you want to be dead for?"

The Janssen kid couldn't meet his eyes, and when he spoke his voice cracked. "Like you said, pop, peace. A little peace of mind, a little quiet. Nobody yammering at you all the time. I mean, if you're dead there's always the chance somebody'll mourn, right? Make friends with the worms, dig their side of it, maybe a little poltergeist action, who knows? I mean, what's the sense of talking about it, anyway? Didn't any of you guys ever just want to run away?"

"Sure thing," said Callahan. "Sometimes I do it too. But I generally run someplace I can find my way back from." It was said so gently that the kid couldn't take offense, though he tried.

"Run away from what, son?" asked Slippery Joe.

The kid had been bottled up tight too long; he exploded. "From what?" he yelled. "Jesus, where do I start? There was this war they wanted me to go and fight, see? And there's this place called college, I mean they want you to care, dig it, care about this education trip, and they don't care enough themselves to make it as attractive as the crap game across the street. There's this air I hear is unfit to breathe, and water that ain't fit to drink, and food that wouldn't nourish a vulture and a grand outlook for the future. You can't get to a job without the car you couldn't afford to run even if you were working, and if you found a job, it'd pay five dollars less than the rent. The T.V. advertises karate classes for four-year-olds and up, the President's New Clothes didn't wear very well, the next depression's around the corner and you ask me what in the name of God I'm running for?

"Man, I've been straight for seven months, what I mean, and in that seven god damned months I have been over this island like a fungus and there is nothing for me. No jobs, no friends, no place to live long enough to get the floor dirty, no money and nobody that doesn't point and say 'Junkie' when I go by for seven months and you ask me what am I running from? Man, everything is all, just everything."

It was right then that I noticed that guy in the corner, the one with the eyes. Remember him? He was leaning forward in rapt attention, his mouth a black slash in a face pulled tight as a drumhead. Those ghastly eyes of his never left the Janssen kid, but somehow I was sure that his awareness included all of us, everyone in the room.

And no one had an answer for the Janssen boy. I could see, all around the room, men who had learned to listen at Callahan's Place, men who had learned to empathize, to want to understand and share the pain of another. And no one had a word to say. They were thinking past the blurted words of a haunted boy, wondering if this crazy world of confusion might not after all be one holy hell of a place to grow up. Most of them already had reason to know damn well that society never forgives the sinner, but they were realizing to their dismay how thin and uncomforting the straight and narrow has become these last few years.

Sure, they'd heard these things before, often enough to make them into clichés. But now I could see the boys reflecting that these were the clichés that made a young man say he liked to feel dead, and the same thought was mirrored on the face of each of them: My God, when did we let these things become clichés? The Problems of Today's Youth were no longer a Sunday supplement or a news broadcast or anything so remote and intangible, they were suddenly become a dirty, shivering boy who told us that in this world we had built for him with our sweat and our blood he was not only tired of living, but so unscared of dying that he did it daily, sometimes, for recreation.

And silence held court in Callahan's Place. No one had a single thing to say, and that guy with the eyes seemed to know it, and to derive some crazy kind of bitter inner satisfaction from the knowledge. He started to settle back in his chair, when Callahan broke the silence.

"So run," he said.

Just like that, flat, no expression, just, "So run." It hung there for about ten seconds, while he and the kid locked eyes.

The kid's forehead started to bead with sweat. Slowly, with shaking fingers, he reached under his leather vest to his shirt pocket. Knuckles white, he hauled out a flat shiny black case about four inches by two. His eyes never left Callahan's as he opened it and held it up so that we could all see the gleaming hypodermic. It didn't look like it had ever been used; he must have just stolen it.

He held it up to the light for a moment, looking up his bare, unmarked arm at it, and then he whirled and flung it case and all into the giant fireplace. Almost as it shattered he sent a cellophane bag of white powder after it, and the powder burned green while the sudden stillness hung in the air. The guy with the eyes looked oddly stricken in some interior way, and he sat absolutely rigid in his seat.

And Callahan was around the bar in an instant, handing the Janssen kid a beer that grew out of his fist and roaring, "Welcome home, Tommy!" and no one in the place was very startled to realize that only Callahan of all of us knew the kid's first name.

We all sort of swarmed around then and swatted the kid on the arm some and he even cried a little until we poured some beer over his head and pretty soon it began to look like the night was going to get merry again after all.

And that's when the guy with eyes stood up, and everybody in the joint shut up and turned to look at him. That sounds melodramatic, but it's the effect he had on us. When he moved, he was the center of attention. He was tall, unreasonably tall, near seven foot, and I'll never know why we hadn't all noticed him right off. He was dressed in a black suit that fit worse than a Joliet Special, and his shoes didn't look right either. After a moment you realized that he had the left shoe on the right foot, and vice-versa, but it didn't surprise you. He was thin and deeply tanned and his mouth was twisted up tight but mostly he was eyes, and I still dream of those eyes and wake up sweating now and again. They were like windows into hell, the very personal and private hell of a man faced with a dilemma he cannot resolve. They did not blink, not once.

He shambled to the bar, and something was wrong with his walk, too, like he was walking sideways on the wall with magnetic shoes and hadn't quite caught the knack yet. He took ten new singles out of his jacket pocket—which struck me as an odd place to keep cash—and laid them on the bar.

Callahan seemed to come back from a place, and hustled around behind the bar again. He looked the stranger up and down and then placed ten shot glasses on the counter. He filled each with rye and stood back silently, running a big red hand through his thinning hair and regarding the stranger with clinical interest.

The dark giant tossed off the first shot, shuffled to the chalk line, and said in oddly-accented English, "To my profession," and hurled the glass into the fireplace.

Then he walked back to the bar and repeated the entire procedure. Ten times.

By the last glass, brick was chipping in the fireplace.

When the last, "To my profession," echoed in empty air, he turned and faced us. He waited, tensely, for question or challenge. There was none. He half turned away, paused, then swung back and took a couple of deep breaths. When he spoke his voice made you hurt to hear it.

"My profession, gentlemen," he said with that funny accent I couldn't place, "is that of advance scout. For a race whose home is many light-years from here. Many, many light-years from here." He paused, looking for our reactions.

Well, I thought, ten whiskeys and he's a Martian. Indeed. Pleased to meet you. I'm Popeye the Sailor. I guess it was pretty obvious we were all thinking the same way, because he looked tired and said, "It would take far more ethanol than that to befuddle me, gentlemen." Nobody said a word to that, and he turned to Callahan. "You know I am not intoxicated," he stated.

Callahan considered him professionally and said finally, "Nope. You're not tight. I'll be a son of a bitch, but you're not tight."

The stranger nodded thanks, spoke thereafter directly to Callahan. "I am here now three days. In two hours I shall be finished. When I am finished I shall go home. After I have gone your planet will be vaporized. I have accumulated data which will ensure the annihilation of your species when they are assimilated by my Masters. To them, you will seem as cancerous cells, in danger of infecting all you touch. You will not be permitted to exist. You will be cured. And I repent me of my profession."

Maybe I wouldn't have believed it anywhere else. But at Callahan's Place anything can happen. Hell, we all believed him. Fast Eddie sang out, "Anyt'ing we can do about it?" and he was serious for sure. You can tell with Fast Eddie.

"I am helpless," the giant alien said dispassionately. "I contain . . . installations . . . which are beyond my influencing—or yours. They have recorded all the data I have perceived in these three days; in two hours a preset mechanism will be triggered and will transmit their contents to the Masters." I looked at my watch: it was eleven-fifteen. "The conclusions of the Masters are foregone. I cannot prevent the transmission; I cannot even attempt to. I am counterprogrammed."

"Why are you in this line of work if it bugs you so much?" Callahan wanted to know. No hostility, no panic. He was trying to understand.

"I am accustomed to take pride in my work," the alien said. "I make safe the paths of the Masters. They must not be threatened by warlike species. I go before, to identify danger, and see to its neutralization. It is a good profession, I think. I thought."

"What changed your mind?" asked Doc Webster sympathetically.

"This place, this . . . 'bar' place we are in—this is not like the rest I have seen. Outside are hatred, competition, morals elevated to the status of ethics, prejudices elevated to the status of morals, whims elevated to the status of prejudices, all things with which I am wearily familiar, the classic symptoms of disease.

"But here is difference. Here in this place I sense qualities, attributes I did not know your species possessed, attributes which everywhere else in the known universe are mutually exclusive of the things I have perceived here tonight. They are good things . . . they cause me great anguish for your passing. They fill me with hurt.

"Oh, that I might lay down my geas," he cried. "I did not know that you had love!"

In the echoing stillness, Callahan said simply, "Sure we do, son. It's mebbe spread a little thin these days, but we've got it all right. Sure would be a shame if it all went up in smoke." He looked down at the rye bottle he still held in his big hand, and absently drank off a couple ounces. "Any chance that your masters might feel the same way?"

"None. Even I can still see that you must be destroyed if the Masters are to be safe. But for the first time in some thousands of years, I regret my profession. I fear I can do no more."

"No way you can gum up the works?"

"None. So long as I am alive and conscious, the transmission will take place. I could not assemble the volition to stop it. I have said: I am counterprogrammed."

I saw Noah Gonzalez's expression soften, heard him say, "Geez, buddy, that's hard lines." A mumbled agreement rose, and Callahan nodded slowly.

"That's tough, brother. I wouldn't want to be in your shoes."

He looked at us with absolute astonishment, the hurt in those terrible eyes of his mixed now with bewilderment. Shorty handed him another drink and it was like he didn't know what to do with it.

"You tell us how much it will take, mister," Shorty said respectfully, "and we'll get you drunk."

The tall man with star-burned skin groaned from deep within himself and backed away until the fireplace contained him. He and the flames ignored each other, and no one found it surprising.

"What is your matter?" he cried. "Why are you not destroying me? You fools, you need only destroy me and you are saved. I am your judge. I am your jury. I will be your executioner."

"You didn't ask for the job," Shorty said gently. "It ain't your doing."

"But you do not understand! If my data are not transmitted, the Masters will assume my destruction and avoid the system forever. Only the equal or superior of a Master could overcome my defenses, but I can control them. I will not use them. Do you comprehend me? I will not activate my defenses—you can destroy me and save yourselves and your species, and I will not hinder you.

"Kill me!" he shrieked.

There was a long, long pause, maybe a second or two, and then Callahan pointed to the drink Shorty still held out and growled, "You better drink that, friend. You need it. Talkin' of killin' in my joint. Wash your mouth out with bourbon and get outta that fireplace, I want to use it."

"Yeah, me too!" came the cry on all sides, and the big guy looked like he was gonna cry. Conversations started up again and Fast Eddie began playing "I Don't Want to Set the World On Fire," in very bad taste indeed.

Some of the boys wandered thoughtfully out, going home to tell their families, or settle their affairs. The rest of us, lacking either concern, drifted over to console the alien. I mean, where else would I want to be on Judgement Day?

He was sitting down, now, with booze of all kinds on the table before him. He looked up at us like a wounded giant. But none of us knew how to begin, and Callahan spoke first.

"You never did tell us your name, friend."

The alien looked startled, and he sat absolutely still, rigid as a fence post, for a long, long moment. His face twisted up awful, as though he was waging some titanic inner battle with himself, and cords of muscle stood up on his neck in what didn't seem to be the right places. Doc Webster began to talk to himself softly.

Then the alien went all blue and shivered like a steel cable under strain, and very suddenly relaxed all over with an audible gasp. He twitched his shoulders experimentally a few times, like he was making sure they were still there, and then he turned to Callahan and said, clear as a bell, "My name is Michael Finn."

It hung in the air for a very long time, while we all stood petrified, suspended.

Then Callahan's face split in a wide grin, and he bellowed, "Why of course! Why yes, yes of course, Mickey Finn. I didn't recognize you for a moment, Mr. Finn," as he trotted behind the bar. His big hands worked busily beneath the counter, and as he emerged with a tall glass of dark fluid the last of us got it. We made way eagerly as Callahan set the glass down before the alien, and stood back with the utmost deference and respect.

He regarded us for a moment, and to see his eyes now was to feel warm and proud. For all the despair and guilt and anguish and horror and most of all the hopelessness were gone from them now, and they were just eyes. Just like yours and mine.

Then he raised his glass and waited, and we all drank with him. Before the last glass was empty his head hit the table like an anvil, and we had to pick him up and carry him to the back room where Callahan keeps a cot, and you know, he was heavy.

And he snored in three stages.

From *Callahan's Crosstime Saloon* by Spider Robinson, 1977. New York: TOR, pp. 1–16.

For good or ill, the mantle of "Interpreter of Ireland to Anglo-American Audiences"
has shifted from James Joyce to Frank McCourt. Here he describes that important Irish
rite of passage, the first pint in a pub.

Angela's Ashes

Frank McCourt

I don't know why Mrs. O'Connell had to shame me before the whole world, and I don't think I'm too good for the post office or anything else. How could I with my hair sticking up, pimples dotting my face, my eyes red and oozing yellow, my teeth crumbling with the rot, no shoulders, no flesh on my arse after cycling thirteen thousand miles to deliver twenty thousand telegrams to every door in Limerick and regions beyond?

Mrs. O'Connell said a long time ago she knew everything about every telegram boy. She must know about the times I went at myself on top of Carrigogunnell, milkmaids gawking, little boys looking up.

She must know about Theresa Carmody and the green sofa, how I got her into a state of sin and sent her to hell, the worst sin of all, worse than Carrigogunnell a thousand times. She must know I never went to confession after Theresa, that I'm doomed to hell myself.

A person that commits a sin like that is never too good for the post office or anything else.

The barman at South's remembers me from the time I sat with Mr. Hannon, Bill Galvin, Uncle Pa Keating, black white black. He remembers my father, how he spent his wages and his dole while singing patriotic songs and making speeches from the dock like a condemned rebel.

And what is it you'd like? says the barman.

I'm here to meet Uncle Pa Keating and have my first pint.

Oh, begod, is that a fact? He'll be here in a minute and sure there's no reason why I shouldn't draw his pint and maybe draw your first pint, is there now?

There isn't, sir.

Uncle Pa comes in and tells me sit next to him against the wall. The barman brings the pints, Uncle Pa pays, lifts his glass, tells the men in the pub, This is my nephew, Frankie McCourt, son of Angela Sheehan, the sister of my wife, having his first pint, here's to your health and long life, Frankie, may you live to enjoy the pint but not too much.

The men lift their pints, nod, drink, and there are creamy lines on their lips and mustaches. I take a great gulp of my pint and Uncle Pa tells me, Slow down for the love o'Jasus, don't drink it all, there's more where that came from as long as the Guinness family stays strong and healthy.

I tell him I want to stand him a pint with my last wages from the post office but he says, No, take the money home to your mother and you can stand me a pint when you come home from America flushed with success and the heat from a blonde hanging on your arm.

The men in the pub are talking about the terrible state of the world and how in God's name Hermann Goering escaped the hangman an hour before the hanging. The Yanks are over there in Nuremberg declaring they don't know how the Nazi bastard hid that pill. Was it in his ear? Up his nostril? Up his arse? Surely the Yanks looked in every hole and cranny of every Nazi they captured and still Hermann wiped their eye. There you are. It shows you can sail across the Atlantic, land in Normandy, bomb Germany off the face of the earth, but when all's said and done they can't find a little pill planted in the far reaches of Goering's fat arse.

Uncle Pa buys me another pint. It's harder to drink because it fills me and makes my belly bulge. The men are talking about concentration camps and the poor Jews that never harmed a soul, men, women, children crammed into ovens, children, mind you, what harm could they do, little shoes scattered everywhere, crammed in, and the pub is misty and the voices fading in and out. Uncle Pa says, Are you all right? You're as white as a sheet. He takes me to the lavatory and the two of us have a good long piss against the wall which keeps moving back and forth. I can't go into the pub again, cigarette smoke, stale Guinness, Goering's fat arse, small shoes scattered, can't go in again, good night, Uncle Pa, thanks, and he tells me go straight home to my mother, straight home, oh, he doesn't know about the excitement on the green sofa or me in such a state of doom that if I died now I'd be in hell in a wink.

Uncle Pa goes back to his pint. I'm out on O'Connell Street and why shouldn't I take the few steps to the Jesuits and tell all my sins this last night I'll be fifteen. I ring the bell at the priests' house and a big man answers, Yes? I tell him, I want to go to confession, Father. He says, I'm not a priest. Don't call me father. I'm a brother.

All right, Brother. I want to go to confession before I'm sixteen tomorrow. State o' grace on my birthday.

He says, Go away. You're drunk. Child like you drunk as a lord ringing for a priest at this hour. Go away or I'll call the guards.

Ah, don't. Ah don't. I only want to go to confession. I'm doomed.

You're drunk and you're not in a proper spirit of repentance.

He closes the door in my face. Another door closed in the face, but I'm sixteen tomorrow and I ring again. The brother opens the door, swings me around, kicks my arse and sends me tripping down the steps.

He says, Ring this bell again and I'll break your hand.

Jesuit brothers are not supposed to talk like that. They're supposed to be like Our Lord, not walking the world threatening people's hands.

I'm dizzy. I'll go home to bed. I hold on to railings along Barrington Street and keep to the wall going down the lane. Mam is by the fire smoking a Woodbine, my brothers upstairs in the bed. She says, That's a nice state to come home in.

It's hard to talk but I tell her I had my first pint with Uncle Pa. No father to get me the first pint.

Your Uncle Pa should know better.

I stagger to a chair and she says, Just like your father.

I try to control the way my tongue moves in my mouth. I'd rather be, I'd rather, rather be like my father than Laman Griffin.

She turns away from me and looks into the ashes in the range but I won't leave her alone because I had my pint, two pints, and I'm sixteen tomorrow, a man.

Did you hear me? I'd rather be like my father than Laman Griffin.

She stands up and faces me. Mind your tongue, she says.

Mind your own bloody tongue.

Don't talk to me like that. I'm your mother.

I'll talk to you any bloody way I like.

You have a mouth like a messenger boy.

Do I? Do I? Well, I'd rather be a messenger boy than the likes of Laman Griffin oul' drunkard with the snotty nose and his loft and people climbing up there with him.

She walks away from me and I follow her upstairs to the small room. She turns, Leave me alone, leave me alone, and I keep barking at her, Laman Griffin, Laman Griffin, till she pushes me, Get out of this room, and I slap her on the cheek so that tears jump in her eyes and there's a small whimpering sound from her, you'll never have the chance to do that again, and I back away from her because there's another sin on my long list and I'm ashamed of myself.

I fall into my bed, clothes and all, and wake up in the middle of the night puking on my pillow, my brothers complaining of the stink, telling me clean up, I'm a disgrace. I hear my mother crying and I want to tell her I'm sorry but why should I after what she did with Laman Griffin.

In the morning my small brothers are gone to school, Malchy is out looking for a job, Mam is at the fire drinking tea. I place my wages on the table by her elbow and turn to go. She says, Do you want a cup of tea?

No.

'Tis your birthday.

I don't care.

She calls up the lane after me, You should have something in your stomach, but I give her my back and turn the corner without answering. I still want to tell her I'm sorry but if I do I'll want to tell her she's the cause of it all, that she should not have climbed to the loft that night and I don't give a fiddler's fart anyway because I'm still writing threatening letters for Mrs. Finucane and saving to go to America.

I have the whole day before I go to Mrs. Finucane to write the threatening letters and I wander down Henry Street till the rain drives me into the Franciscan church where St. Francis stands with his birds and lambs. I look at him and wonder why I ever prayed to him. No, I didn't pray, I begged.

I begged him to intercede for Theresa Carmody but he never did a thing, stood up there on his pedestal with the little smile, the birds, the lambs, and didn't give a fiddler's fart about Theresa or me.

I'm finished with you, St. Francis. Moving on. Francis. I don't know why they ever gave me that name. I'd be better off if they called me Malachy, one a king, the other a great saint. Why didn't you heal Theresa? Why did you let her go to hell? You let my mother climb to the loft. You let me get into a state of doom. Little children's shoes scattered in concentration camps. I have the abscess again. It's in my chest and I'm hungry.

St. Francis is no help, he won't stop the tears bursting out of my two eyes, the sniffling and choking and the God oh Gods that have me on my knees with my head on the back of the pew before me and I'm so weak with the hunger and the crying I could fall on the floor and would you please help me God or St. Francis because I'm sixteen today and I hit my mother and sent Theresa to hell and wanked all over Limerick and the county beyond I dread the millstone around my neck.

There is an arm around my shoulders, a brown robe, click of black rosary beads, a Franciscan priest.

My child, my child, my child.

I'm a child and I lean against him, little Frankie on his father's lap, tell me all about Cuchulain, Dad, my story that Malachy can't have or Freddie Leibowitz on swings.

My child, sit here with me. Tell me what troubles you. Only if you want to. I am Father Gregory.

I'm sixteen today, Father.

Oh, lovely, lovely, and why should that be a trouble to you?

I drank my first pint last night.

Yes?

I hit my mother.

God help us, my child. But He will forgive you. Is there anything else?

I can't tell you, Father.

Would you like to go to confession?

I can't, Father. I did terrible things.

God forgives all who repent. He sent His only Beloved Son to die for us.

I can't tell, Father. I can't.

But you could tell St. Francis, couldn't you?

He doesn't help me anymore.

But you love him, don't you?

I do. My name is Francis.

Then tell him. We'll sit here and you'll tell him the things that trouble you. If I sit and listen it will only be a pair of ears for St. Francis and Our Lord. Won't that help?

I talk to St. Francis and tell him about Margaret, Oliver, Eugene, my father singing Roddy McCorley and bringing home no money, my father sending no money from England, Theresa and the green sofa, my terrible sins on Carrigogunnell, why couldn't they hang Hermann Goering for what he did to the little children with shoes scattered around concentration camps, the Christian Brother who closed the

FRANK McCOURT

door in my face, the time they wouldn't let me be an altar boy, my small brother Michael walking up the lane with the broken shoe clacking, my bad eyes that I'm ashamed of, the Jesuit brother who closed the door in my face, the tears in Mam's eyes when I slapped her.

Father Gregory says, Would you like to sit and be silent, perhaps pray for a few minutes?

His brown robe is rough against my cheek and there's a smell of soap. He looks at St. Francis and the tabernacle and nods and I suppose he's talking to God. Then he tells me kneel, gives me absolution, tells me say three Hail Marys, three Our Fathers, three Glory Bes. He tells me God forgives me and I must forgive myself, that God loves me and I must love myself for only when you love God in yourself can you love all God's creatures.

But I want to know about Theresa Carmody in hell, Father.

No, my child. She is surely in heaven. She suffered like the martyrs in olden times and God knows that's penance enough. You can be sure the sisters in the hospital didn't let her die without a priest.

Are you sure, Father?

I am, my child.

He blesses me again, asks me to pray for him, and I'm happy trotting through the rainy streets of Limerick knowing Theresa is in heaven with the cough gone.

Nora Lane is the pseudonym of a screenwriter and poetess in the Los Angeles area. Her father was a noted fixture on the New York literary scene from the 1920s to the '60s. Here she reminisces about his drinking with a few then-celebrities.

The Wine of Life

Nora Lane

"Come fill the cup"
"The wine of life keeps oozing drop by drop"
"And the lord changed the water into wine"

Poetic and biblical references raise booze to a high plateau. Man, the predator, abuses it. Now it is regarded as the forerunner of violent crimes, as the reason cars crash into one another, causing death. Formerly, it was the drink of kings and queens, the co-habiter of the civilized.

Let's go back a frame. Here is a writer at work, his typewriter his tool. He knows Mencken. Does articles for the *Mercury,* short stories for *The New Yorker,* commentary pieces for the *Commonweal,* and so many others. He likes Hearst. When he was young, and working for Hearst, this writer referred to him as the "Old Man." Old Man Hearst was loved by those he had scouted and brought to work for him. He had found the writer at Harvard University. Hearst promoted yellow journalism, the confidential of that era; exposé, scandal. It was a day when a writer could do no wrong, before the laws came in and limited their power.

His last born, a girl he calls Tisha, is watching, solemn-eyed. Fifty years old at her birth, he is now looking at life with different eyes—remembering how he was discovered as a cub reporter. Ah, those were the days of free flowing booze, and absolute freedom for writers. Today is special, Tisha's seventh birthday. As a treat, daddy is taking her to those places he frequents. Places where writers and poets exchange ideas, anecdotes. What is going on in the writing game!

Mother is waiting to be kissed good-bye. A classical violinist, she played violin in elegant hotels before she met daddy. A beautiful girl, long red hair. She caught the attention of an older man, Marlon Brando Senior. He wrote love poems and placed them on the seat where she was playing. She never dated him. Her father, Samuel Winfield Priest Arnold, was a wealthy man, and related to many of the best families in the South. Until the Stock Market Crash.

It's time. Let's go. We are off. Wait! It's only 5 A.M. Daddy is making coffee. He is standing there, black hair, green eyes, a face red from exposure, drinking. Not booze, coffee. He is doing his navy exercises, push-ups. I stand by. I am the watcher. I am on a trip where grown-ups will look at me, and expect me to say something wise because daddy is a genius. At last, it is time.

Daddy smiles at me, we are in a cab. Daddy is always in a suit and tie, though it is summer in New York. I look out the window as daddy and the cabby talk. New York is cleaning up from the previous night's spillage. The city seems to sparkle with excitement. The ride ends. Daddy lifts me out. I don't like that. I'm not a baby. We enter Julius's. A place where artists, writers, and poets hang. Some wannabes, some realities mingle, bonded together by a mutual obsession: art. We are sitting at a rickety table near the door. The floor is covered with sawdust, a man at the bar is yodeling. Some give him money. Others applaud. I see these people are not us. Men in jeans and T-shirts, women in cotton. Then I ask daddy if I can have a drink. He goes to the bar and brings me what looks like a lemonade. I try to hide my disappointment. The drink is sweet, but there is something else. A dash of claret wine. I'm watching the door. It opens. A man in a suit and a tie. He is a friend. This is the George that daddy promised. George Putnam. I run to him, kiss him happily. His face is a cold mask. I am crushed. And I tell him so. He smiles, assures me it's him, not me. A bird he loved and lost left the nest. Her name, Lee Carson. In a place where deep love is rare. This is like an old time movie. Daddy is playing the role of consoler. It's new to him, but he is doing well, as George is laughing. I am attracted to the tragedy of his love. I think I will play this role myself, when I become the great actress everyone predicts. George comes from a wordy family. They are publishers. He is a talker. Makes me want to grow up quickly. George asks about school. I say it's great. He wants the waiter to bring me a birthday cake. Daddy says no. It's an at-home celebration. The men are drinking Scotch. My claret lemonade is beginning to pall. I make a face and want to ask daddy for a coke but they are in deep conversation. I dare not interrupt, although a lot of time has gone by. At last, we thank George and wave good-bye. George stays to talk to the bartender. I like him.

On our way to our next appointment, daddy is getting into what mother calls his silly mood. He is speaking to the cabby in New Yorkese. He is good at it. Were he not a writer, I believe he would be a fine actor. He has kind of a Barrymore nose but not quite. Daddy and the cabby are pals now. The cabby points out a raggedy lady clutching a wine bottle. She is holding it tightly against a bony, bare chest and looking daggers at us. We cruise by slowly and she points an angry finger at us and spits. The sputum lands not on the cab but on a man wearing a black tee-shirt. He does not stop, makes a face, shakes his fist at the woman and runs across the street. The cabby lifts his hat in salute. To the woman or her victim, I do not know.

We arrive twenty minutes late. George Hamilton Combs is going on the air in twenty minutes. He fluffs off daddy's apology as though it is unimportant. Twenty minutes. So daddy and he must reacquaint themselves rapidly. Combs apologizes for what he calls his rum blossom. He explains that it is a strange thing. The blossom appears when he goes over his five drink limit. As if he is being punished. He and daddy discuss the possible psychological element and laugh. He invites us to the show. His blue eyes are so friendly and his socialite wife wants to meet daddy because of a short story he wrote for the *New Yorker* that she just loved. Daddy regrets, says we can't make because of our next appointment. They promise to be in touch. We wave good-bye, and on to the next George.

Daddy is laughing, waxing poetic in the cab, reciting Poe's "Raven" and "The Bells." Night after night, when I go to bed unable to sleep, daddy reads Poe's short stories and poems to me. I generally nod off when the he reads "The Bells." But now daddy is boasting to the big burly driver that none of his literary circle of friends were ever arrested for drunk driving. He says it's because they have the best designated drivers—New York cabbies. The driver chuckles.

We track the third George down to Eddie Condon's Jazz Club. We go to the wrong address. At last, rerouted, we are seated at a table near the bandstand. Georges Brunis is a short, fat man from New Orleans. He is sitting with us, swilling gin at a rapid pace. A beautiful *Vogue* model comes to our table and insists on dragging Georges away. He apologizes. She is dressed in red chiffon and has black hair twisted into a chignon. A perfect face. She takes him outside for a private conversation. Georges comes back laughing. Daddy says, "what a beautiful girl!" Georges answers that she is too thin and greedy. He and daddy talk about Storyville, where Georges got his start playing at age fourteen.

As the set begins, Georges jumps onto the stage, the spotlight on him, as he sings the *Song of the Bayou,*—"Oh Lord, please take away the darkness!"—soul music. The trombone sounds like pain itself, mournful. Tears are flowing from old, tired eyes. Men remembering when it was all perfect, before the road came in, as they say. Georges is pounding out another song, "Ugly Child." Georges is totally fascinating. His eyes, dark brown, are long, almost to his ears. Oily skin, pock marked with jasmine perfume spread on his kinky gray hair. We shout, to be heard above the applause, "Das V'ddanya!" I ask daddy to tell me about this man, why people are drawn to him. Daddy says he comes from the most exciting town in the U.S. His mother, father, entire family are musicians; each one lost in music. They are not from the staid world that we live in.

The frame fades—it is the present once more.

Don't hate booze. The shy come out of their shell and shout. It brings people together. No offense to MADD, they have their own tragic agenda. But, if we insist, as they do, that not even one drink is allowed on the road, because of an altered personality, then we must outlaw aspirin, stress pills, anti-depressants—even automobiles themselves. So, to your health and mine.

One of the great thrills of the drinking life is finding a semi-secret and illegal bar, where the drinks are good and the place unregulated. Here is one such phantom tavern. Located in L.A., it could be in any of our major cities.

The Joss Bar

Jeremy Rosenberg

"The Shipwreck: Banana, coconut, papaya, rum. You won't know what hit you, but you'll suddenly find yourself ashore."

Jack Dallas[1] stands behind the homemade and heavily bamboo'd bar in his 400-square-foot Hollywood efficiency. Pours a drink. "You won't know what hit you," Dallas says, "but you'll suddenly find yourself ashore." This is Dallas' joint. Booze mecca. No charge. Open bar. No secret knocks. No passwords. Calls it Joss Bar, after the paper polyurethaned to the flat drink mantle. Joss, the same paper burned at Chinese funerals.

The place is twenty by twenty feet. Bathroom and closet to one side, with a partial wall. Kitchen on other side. In the greater middle plane, a rectangle. One corner clipped off for computer, phone and drawing table. Most obscured by bamboo and brocade three-panel Chinese folding screen. More of the panda produce throughout. Blow-dart-gun-thin reeds.

Up above the bar is a thatched hut roof that looks like brown sunkist blonde layered hair of a surfer. A seaside shack in Mexico. Shuffleboard court in Florida.

"I wanted to design a space where I would feel comfortable," Dallas says. "I chose bamboo. Everything else just filtered in."

Fish nets hang from ceiling, cast shadows like topographic maps.

The wall behind the bar is covered with cross-hatched grass matting, squishy to the touch. Like a bird's nest, from egg's view.

Here are two skulls. Plastic. One flips open, mango candies inside. An alligator

---

1. Jack Dallas is the legal doing business as, but not given name of, a Los Angeles resident.

head, from a Bayou curio shop. Theosophy poster. Kreskin's ESP, a parlor game. An acupuncture model, diagramming pressure points.

Oh yeah, the bed. Folded up into futon sofa. The desk, computer, telephone. Pads and sketchbooks. Easel.

Dallas lives here, paints here. Hosts and bartends here.

And this is Dallas. White dude. Clean shaven. Thirty? Thirty-five? Maybe younger. Ex-military. Okinawa, six months. Won't ever say more. Has family connections with the secrets and sauce. Great-grandma was a moonshiner, made bathtub gin in Prohibition-era Chicago. Po's raided once, saw poverty, winked mercy. Said kill the still but made no arrest. Great-grandma went right on cooking.

Dallas, at his joint. Holds court. Murray's Pomade in brown hair. Apply with two palms, push strands up, then smooth back. Wears shortsleeved shirts, silks or blends. Most gatherings, flies the Guayabera, flame red gear, popular in warm-weather locales. The Philippines. Made in Korea. Dallas removed the pockets. Nothing to hide.

"The Icy Tarmac: Frosted vodka plus licorice. One or two of those, you'll be happy to slide into somebody."

Dallas makes calls. Invites twenty over, female and male. That's what the room can hold. Animators. Crafters. Writers. Treats them to concoctions. Guests sit on two bar stools, pair of other chairs, and on his futon, the one with the furry gray cover that feels like a rabbit's hide and looks like an elephant's.

The visitors chat. His age and younger. Look down, on the old steamer trunk with the buckles and snaps. See Hush-Hush. Gossip rag from the '40s. Sample headlines:

"Exposed: The $300,000,000 Davy Crockett Racket."

"The Naked Truth about Terry Moore's Fantastic Antics."

"The Lowdown: Hedy Lamar's Strange Bout with the Lie Detector."

Mag's a reminder of Dallas' day job. He fields calls, tracks tales for a celebrity journalist. That's new way to say gossip columnist.

Dallas is discrete. Dummies up until publication. Then repeats. The big screen ingenue using the butt double. The '70s singer with such a midnight jones for crack that he smashes the glass stem and smokes the shards.

"It can drive you mad," the barkeep says. "I've heard things that would make your eyes spin."

*   *   *

"The Monkey's Paw: Blended drink. Frothy banana pleasure. You couldn't ask for more, except for an opposable thumb."

Dallas takes the silver mixing tin and the clear glass mixing cup and shakes them back and forth, elbows wide, like Houdini trying to escape a straightjacket.

He pours a green drink into a martini glass. Calls it a Headhunter's Honey. Stirs it with a chopstick held loose like a jazz drummer's brush. Keeps time. Cracks his knuckles, sounds like felled redwood.

Full set list:

Mildred Bailey, throaty jazz singer from the '40s. Charles Trénet, "The Singing Madman," bald, wore a monocle. Famed for acting, looking like a chicken. Tampa Red. Mexican Go-Go tunes. Blues. Rockabilly. Curtis Mayfield. Tom Waits. Trance and electronica.

"The Grassy Knoll: A vodka absinthe equivalent. Kind of like Dallas, 1963—you wonder where the shot is coming from."

You'd never know from the outside. Dallas resides in, pours out of, a three-story brick apartment house thrown up eighty-years-ago. Brick building, ivy covered, some nice in-laid ornamentation. Now on a dead-end cul-de-sac overlooking a freeway.

Dial digits to be buzzed through the metal gate. The wood door, heavy, paint peeling, unlocked. Sign over trough for mail packages reads, "This is not a trash basket." Nearby notice: "Caution, Broken Tile." Big middle chunk of the third step up out of four has crumbled.

The public interior is covered with gray shag. Carpet bespotted, stained like a rummy's liver.

"The only thing that's really notable in this building, besides myself," Dallas says, chuckles, "Is that Elizabeth Short stayed here when it was a residence hotel."

She: The Black Dahlia. Murder. Infamy.

More recently, more trouble. Ten years ago, Dallas hears, the place was a drive-up crack den. Autos pulled up to street level panes, made buys.

These days, there's a senior citizen home across the street.

"Seven Seas Regret. A special mix. Like Malibu dirt—it slides, baby."

Dallas never charges his guests, blows his own sleight dough. Accepts food donations, sometimes hard stuff. Has a candy-color collection, mouthwash-looking menagerie of syrups and mixers and the Sherlock Holmes stuff—the proof. Cherry Flavor brandy. Crème de Noyeaux. Crème de Banana. Blue Curacao. Sour Apple Schnapps. Lychee Punch. Vermouth. Compari. Drambuie. Midori Melon Liquor. Joss is about the soft stuff. That's what pleases the crowd. Toughest guests walk in grizzled. Ask for martinis. See surroundings. Smile. Chips cascade from shoulders. "You can have the biggest bruiser in the world and he's not going to just want beer," Dallas says. "Sooner or later he's going to back down and he's going to want some foofy little apple drink. When you get right down to it, people want to look forward to their drink. They don't want to be punished by it."

Exception:

Has Phoenix brand Gao Ling Chiu, two peacocks on the bottle and an emblem of a monkey. Basically a rice brandy, 112 proof, 56% alcohol. Yellow-clear hue, a la industrial cleaner. Just barely on the edge of blinding, barkeep says. "Drink it straight, it's a lot like drinking paint thinner. It's powerful stuff. It will make you hurt. It'll make it seem like grappa is a soft drink."

And Dallas drinks Macallan scotch when he's alone.

The habit starts to cost. Fifty bottles of exotic booze, always, on a crank job's wages.

Dallas thinks maybe sometimes to come full circle. Open Joss Bar up to strangers with cash, tapping secret knocks on his door. Be like great-grandma with her still. Maybe build bamboo cages for go-go dancers. Hope the po's don't raid. Hope the neighbors keep leaving him alone.

For now, he won't even accept private bartending gigs. Just Joss, free and clear, that's all. Whether it makes any sense or not.

"There are moments," the man says, "When I look around and say, 'What the hell?' Couldn't I just go out and buy a six pack like everybody else?"

Reprinted with permission from the *LA Times Magazine.*

As noted in the Introduction, Nick von Knupffer is a very good friend, with whom I have downed many a drink. But the good Baron does not only imbibe, he appreciates what he imbibes. Here he immortalizes one of his favorite potations.

An Ode to Pimms

Nicholas, Baron von Knupffer

This substance, this addiction, this liquid,
I lose all control of my limbs,
Happiness, colored and vivid,
This substance, this liquid called Pimms.

To imbibe, to absorb, or to drink,
The fruit, the mint, the lemonade,
Not allowing me much but to think,
And to write, it will give me some aid.

As a rival to my great friend the vine,
And the demon itself in Absinthe,
Oh, how I love to drink when I dine,
To descend even deeper to sin.

All alone I remain now awake,
My brothers asleep with no pain,
Not a noise that I dare longer make,
With the Pimms, 'tis death I shall feign.

My dear friend, you will surely be missed,
At the ball where the fair maidens dance,
I am certain we will then get pissed,
And then bugger off south to France.

The gang will not be complete,
Confused, is what Sasha shall think,
This June we were due all to meet,
You, forgiven, absolved by the drink.

As the room now again starts to spin,
My soul now touched by it all,
I learn how corrupt is my kin,
By the great lord, the king Ethanol.

Two by Sugar

Bert Randolph Sugar

DRINKING WITH HEMINGWAY

After a certain period of time, the mind manages to retain the essentials, which means I can tell you this much: somehow, someway, I drank with Ernest Hemingway back in 1956. And what I remember about that moment is cut and restitched to suit my fancy—and my memory, such as it is. The occasion was a term paper for a then— snotnosed college student (me) on those who loomed large in letters—men like Hemingway, Faulkner and O'Hara. Somehow my professor had managed to arrange for me to interview Hemingway, during a layover at Chicago's O'Hare Airport.

Preparing myself to meet the Great Man, I read and reread all of his works and found a recurring thread: most of them contained more than just some mention of drink, many were marinated in the same. Take *The Killers,* for instance. In it he wrote, "Liquor is a Giant Killer and nobody who has not had to deal with the Giant many, many times has any right to speak against the Giant Killer." In many of his other works he would drop in references to drink as a barkeep would an olive in a martini, writing, "In Europe then we thought of wines as something as healthy and normal as food and also as a great river of happiness and well being and delight. Drinking wine was not a snobbism nor a sign of sophistication nor a cult; it was as natural as eating and to me as necessary." Or writing about absinthe: ". . . of all things he had enjoyed and forgotten and that came back to him when he tasted that opaque, bitter, tongue-numbing, brain-warming, stomach-warming, idea-changing liquid alchemy . . ." This all from someone who once said, "Drink all you want, but don't be a drunken shit. I drink and get drunk everyday, but I never bother anyone." Immortal advice, albeit advice the notoriously belligerent Hemingway rarely took himself.

Knowing more than most about the Great Man (surely more than Yogi Berra, who, upon being introduced to Hemingway for the first time by restaurateur Toots Shor, asked, "What paper does he write for?"), I armed myself with questions. Ready to deal them up as if by the heaping plateful, I stood at the gate, waiting for this man whose drinking feats formed an institution, knowing that somehow, someway, we would wind up at a bar. And then there he was, disembarking from his DC 10, down the stairs, passing through the gate and the furnace of what was a boiling July day. Toting a shoulder bag, along with greatness and dignity on his twin shoulders, the bearded man with the safari-like hat and open brown shirt, came striding into the waiting room.

With time too short for a course in etiquette, I hurried up to him, hand extended, and introduced myself—or sputtered something that sounded like an introduction. He looked at my outstretched hand with all the affection one would lavish on widow-and-orphan oppressors with more than a slight tinge of Bright's disease thrown in and then grumbled something about it being "hot as hell," and "Let's find a bar so we can talk." And so, as he wheeled around and set off in search of a bar with the same unerring instincts of a hunting dog on the trail of a pheasant, I paddled along behind him, trying to make conversation but merely talking to his back. Finally, after about a five-minute walk, our destination was in sight, and he quickened his pace, arriving at a barstool that looked like it had his name on it less than two ticks of the small hand of the clock from its first coming into view. Knowing that time was too short and that I had the Great Man's company—if not his attention, which was now focused on hailing the barkeep and ordering what he called "a highball"—I began to ask him questions.

Quickly I found that asking him about F. Scott Fitzgerald was like asking a lamp post how it felt about dogs, an opinion he grunted between swigs of his highball before, in less time than it takes to read this, slamming it back on the bar and asking for another. What I didn't learn about Fitzgerald, however, I soon learned about drinks. And drinking. Out came: "Never delay kissing a pretty girl or opening a bottle of whiskey," as he downed his third highball. Then, staring at the bottom of his glass, he said, almost under his breath, "I decided to stop drinking with creeps, and I decided to drink only with friends. I've lost thirty pounds . . ." Or something that sounded like that which sounded as if it came from one of his works, although I wasn't sure which one. Then, talking about the many places he had been, and many places he had been at one with alcohol, he allowed something I've taken as gospel to this day: there was not only a drink for all seasons, but all reasons and all residences. "A Martinique rum," he said by way of example, "is the perfect antidote for a rainy day." Or somesuch.

Now, I would like to be clearer in my recollections. However, by this time, I was on the verge of collapsing like a balloon with the string suddenly unattached—his drinking style such that it made great demands upon his companion. And I, having decided to attempt to keep up with the Great Man on a one-on-one basis, was beginning to feel powers barely those of respiration. What else do I remember about our discussion? Here I must tell you that his interest was less in conversation with the youngster at his elbow than with throwing his drinks off faster than a snake sheds his skin. His next flight was to take him to a hunt somewhere in Idaho. Or was it Montana? Who the hell knew by this time? He also said, I think, something about Gertrude Stein and the origin of her famous phrase, "The Lost Generation," saying that it had been uttered while she waited for some particularly inept French mechanic to fix her Model T and the owner of the garage had said to the mechanic, "You are all a generation perdue," which became, in translation, "A lost generation."

Finally, after two or three more highballs, this Mona Lisa of modern literature slammed his (again) empty glass down on the bar, and with manners hardly overcharged with courtesy, said something that sounded like "Good bye" and strode off, leaving me to pay the bill. I reflected on what had just taken place. I had notes that would have to wait for future cryptographers to decode, a headache that made my head feel as if it were ready for mounting on Mount Rushmore and a bill I had been stuck with. All in all, a small price to have had a drink, or eight, with Hemingway. Or was that the past tense—had a *drunk* with Hemingway?

THE BAR EXAM

As someone who has reached that stage in a long drinking career where he believes being a good liver is better than having one, I came to look upon this assignment as not only an award for life well spent, but also as one of the best pieces of type-casting since Milton Berle played himself in Broadway Danny Rose. After all, I basically began researching this story when Father Adam first heard the stampede of the apple cider salesman, and I haven't slowed down since.

Still, I reasoned, you can't know enough about your subject. That, and the fact that the alcohol level in my blood had fallen to a dangerously low level, propelled me in the direction of one of my favorite watering holes, O'Lunney's, just off Times Square in Manhattan, where I could do more research in advance of my Rubaiyat of the Scotch and Soda. Establishing homesteading rights to a bar stool in the corner, all the better to commune with nature and the bottom of my glass, I began to put my thoughts down on the official bar stationery—its napkins. However, it was a train of thought that never quite reached its destination, interrupted as it was by two dues-paying customers who had come in and were now hail-fellowing and swapping stories just this side of wind-baggery. Unable to collect my thoughts, I hurriedly collected my bar napkins that contained them and, bolting out of my stool as if it were incandescent, cut myself away from my original moorings and headed out the exit with migratory ambitions.

My second installment of scenery was Annie Moore's, up the block from O'Lunney's, where I was doing my best imitation of one of Madame Tussaud's waxworks when I was again disturbed, this time by someone whose pneumatic pipe organs punctured whatever idea balloons I had managed to get aloft. And although he was to ask, "May I drive you home?" he already had, as I raced out with something of the wild joy prisoners feel at the announcement of their parole, back to the quiet confines of home where I could have a more pleasant think on the subject of drink.

It was there, comforted by two very old friends of mine, Jack Daniels and Jim Beam, that I began reflecting on the good life of laboring in the backyards and vineyards of saloons. After all this time the mind retains the essential and rejects the superficial—my wife calls it "Cuttysheimers." So when choosing a place to drink, it's perhaps best to start with where not to go.

Rule #1. Never go to a bar that serves umbrellas in your drink or colors your drink. Especially pink.

Rule #2. Never go to a bar that has "happy hour." Nobody there ever is.

Rule #3. Never go to a bar where the bartender has more problems than you do.

Rule #4. Never go to a bar where you raise the average age of those inside by more than five years just by walking in.

Rule #5. Although my favorite pubs are Irish pubs, never go to one on St. Paddy's Day. It's amateur night and a good time to get a reservation at a Chinese restaurant.

Rule #6. Never go to a bar where there is more than one bouncer unless you're expecting the trouble they are.

Rule #7. Never go to a bar where they allow cell phones. A bar is a place of sanctity—check your self-importance at the door.

Rule #8. Never go to a bar that does not ask you what brand you prefer, but instead pours something called "Old Panther Piss" aged in the woods from the well underneath the counter.

Rule #9. Never go to a bar that does not allow cigar smoking. A personal preference, granted, but you should tell anyone who complains, "If it wasn't for twenty cigars a day smoked by Winston Churchill, you'd be speaking German."

Rule #10. Never drive and drink. The world needs designated drivers—and where would they be without designated drunks sitting in the back seat getting sick all over themselves? They'd be out of work, that's where.

That being said, there are as many reasons to frequent bars as there are, well, bars. Most, when asked why they go to a particular bar, will give an answer somewhat akin to Saul Bellow's after he was asked the difference between the words "ignorance" and "indifference": "I don't know and I don't care." But you should—both know and care, for picking the right drinking emporium is all-important. It's almost an art: a lost art at that. Over my well-spent years I have collected good reasons for frequenting saloons and good lessons for picking them like liquor labels on a well-traveled steamer trunk, starting with the very first time I ever bellied up. That bar was across the street from the old Washington Evening Star, where I held the exalted position of part-time gopher and copy boy—a phrase that disappeared into a haze of political correctness in the same way a plane's "cockpit" is now called a "flight deck." I was just fourteen, my face still a stranger to the razor, and I ordered a draft beer. From the very first sip, I was hooked. Not on drink, but on the camaraderie that came with it, the chance to meet those I worked with in more convivial surroundings and swap stories—to share the feeling of "belonging." It was to be the beginning of a life dedicated to one noble pursuit: having the most fun one can have with his clothes on.

It was in just such bars that I would gain an education far beyond that taught in the classrooms of my college life, a college life that went on for nine years and consisted of boosting the liquor agent every time I bent my elbow. Nine years because when my parents divorced, my kindly grandfather put his hand on my shoulder and said, "Don't worry, son, I'll take care of you and send you to college." That, of course, included my mounting bar bills, caused by the many times I mounted a bar stool and ordered Thomases & Jeremiahs, or somesuch. And when he passed on, lo those nine years later, I had to abandon my career as a professional student. (If he were still alive today, very still at the age of 124, I would still be in college.)

But while there, back in those politically incorrect days when men were men and women were damned glad of it, I was able to soak up the many lessons of drinking in the company of my fellow drinking companions, mostly the members of my rugby team. Lessons like: drinking is not a survivor sport; knowing which drinks were user-friendly and not, as Satchel Paige said, "unsettling" to my stomach and head; and how to socialize, both with my own crowd and with others at the bar—many of whom I played bar trivia with, hustling up the unwanted change that was there for the taking and winning more than my share of money. I also won knowledge, about different people and the places they'd been and the jobs they'd held and the characters they'd met. Alas, they never gave me course credits for that, but I learned more in bars than I did in contracts class.

Sometimes, though, the object of my visitation was less bonding with males than bundling with females. Throughout most of those nine years I might just as well have been a member of a Dominican order, but one day I met a young lady with promiscuous ears who just happened to be sitting on the bar stool next to me, as overlooked as Whistler's father. To her, "hello" was an aphrodisiac. I wouldn't have noticed her had it not been for one endearing characteristic: she had Texas-sized measurements, approximately 52-34-44, the other breast being just a little bit smaller. It was lust at first sight. By the end of the evening, my friends were needling me that I now had two ambitions in life: to get a write-up in Life magazine and to get an upright in her.

I had already, I thought, made plans to acquit one of those two goals, scheduling a rendezvous with her over Thanksgiving weekend in New York. I came up from Washington to meet her at the Astor Hotel, at the time considered one of the city's finest, forever memorialized by Frank Sinatra and Bing Crosby in the movie *High Society,* when they sang the line, "Have you heard of Mimsy Starr/She got pinched in the Ass-tor Bar." So there I was, sitting at the Ass-tor Bar, awaiting the opportunity to pinch the fair maiden, when I heard a female voice that struck a familiar chord; it sounded eerily like a voice from the recently released movie *Some Like It Hot.* So I tottered off the stool and walked around to see if my audio identity was correct. And what to my wondering eyes should appear but a vision depriving me of breath and causing my eyeballs to rotate in their parent sockets: Marilyn Monroe.

She looked like she was made of sunshine, blood-red tissue and clear weather, the most beautiful woman I had ever laid eyes on—the operative words here "eyes on," since the other word didn't come into play. And so, after a small stagger at a passable version of the Mother Tongue, I did likewise, staggering out onto Broadway. My date had stood me up, Marilyn had turned me down, and so I voyaged, Columbus-like, in search of other bars and local fauna of the two-legged variety. To make a long story longer—and who ever heard of a short bar story anyway?—when I returned to school after that weekend, I found that the object of my non-affections, good ol' what's-her-name, had in fact shown up at the Astor Bar and, finding me talking to "some blond," had abruptly turned on her high heels and left. I still think I got the best of the bargain.

Never let it be said, however, that the primary reason to frequent a bar is for women. Truth be told, bar time is guy time—a time to argue, wager, commiserate, celebrate, even get a job. The latter was one of my underlying goals after I graduated from law school—I guess you could call it graduating, having finished 313th out of a class of 313. I went on to pass the bar, and, I might say proudly, it was the only bar I ever passed as I continued to go on my merry way, from bar to bar, and city to city, undergoing trial by elbow. For reasons I never quite understood, I had decided to become a sportswriter. I wanted to be another Red Smith, but by the time I found out that I was never going to be, it was too late. So with that ambition in mind and a resume tucked under my arm, I headed to New York.

As any young musician would go directly to Carnegie Hall without passing GO and collecting $200, I now went straight to the place Red Smith called "the mother lode": Toots Shor's. Shor's was where New York's sporting crowd hung out for the meat of this century, a bar for guys' guys, that catered to those who wished to be seen and obscene—the athletes, writers, actors and anyone who was anyone, or wished they were, back in those days. It was always crowded to the gunwales, as it was the night Charlie Chaplin, nervously waiting for a table, complained to Toots about the need to stand in line. Toots paid him no-never-mind, merely shouting over his shoulder, "Just stand there and be funny" to the world's funniest man, who was not in a very funny mood at the moment. Another time, Toots, who was partial to athletes, especially those who played for his favorite team, the New York baseball Giants, was talking to Sir Alexander Fleming. Not exactly sure who it was he was talking to and trying to make polite conversation—which came hard to Toots, his normal dialogue peppered with a cheerful contempt for the English language and words like "crum-bum"—Toots was more than pleased to have one of his waiters come over and tug on his jacket to tell him that Mel Ott, the manager of the Giants, had just come in. Glad for the rescue, Toots merely waved to Sir Alexander, saying "'Scuse me, but somebody important just walked in . . ." and wandered away, leaving the discoverer of penicillin standing there, molding away.

On the afternoon I first bivouacked there, the bar stools were filled with people who looked like they were filling the help-wanted columns more than the sports columns, the stuff of which unsungs were made. But there was one scene going on down at the end of this rather looooong, somewhat circular bar, something that resembled a two-man debating society—it was a drinking contest between Shor and Jackie Gleason.

These two had had all manner of contests before, including their famous run-around-the-block race, with each taking off from the front door of the restaurant in opposite directions down 51st Street—once around the block for fifty dollars. When Toots, huffing and puffing, staggered back to the restaurant, he found Gleason comfortably ensconced at the bar, glass in hand. Toots couldn't believe it. Nor could he believe that he had not seen Gleason pass him going the opposite way as he went around the block. Finally, Gleason let on. He had hired a cab in front of the restaurant and had ridden around the block, leaving Toots to do a solo.

Now they were taking each other on in another contest: a drinking bout. Apparently the bout was one that had been going on since noon, and I was watching its championship rounds. After another two hours, Gleason got up on legs not exactly fulfilling the function they had sworn to uphold and tottered off, presumably to sample the soap in the men's room. However, he never quite made it, falling face down and now doing his best imitation of a beached whale, blocking the entrance to the dining room, leaving no room for any of the patrons to get over, by or around him. Finally, after a period of time in which it was thought the only thing that could improve him was embalming fluid, one concerned waiter came over and asked Toots if he could move him. "Screw him, he's no trooper," growled Toots. "Leave the crumbum where he is." You ain't gonna see that at the local Houlihan's, guys.

Shor's is long gone and the Astor Bar ain't the Ass-tor Bar anymore. But most cities have a few gems left. Granted, over the years bars have changed. Their curriculum is now a more varied one, but still one devoted to the same single-minded orthodoxy: drinking. And its natural extensions, camaraderie and fun.

And over the course of my well-spent drinking life, I've had fun—and more memories than I can press between the pages of my mind. Memories like standing at the Betty Boop Bar at the MGM Grand in Las Vegas and being introduced to Divine Brown, Hugh Grant's old friend, after she became the busiest memory in Hollywood, and her asking me to buy her a Courvoisier. Or spending one evening in a Philadelphia hotel bar with gap-toothed Leon Spinks, the former heavyweight champ as inarticulate as Muhummad Ali was eloquent, at first wondering if there was something wrong with my sense of hearing, but eventually wondering if I was hearing Sir Laurence Olivier deliver the balcony scene from Romeo and Juliet. Or closing a downtown watering hole one night with two members of the pennant-winning Oakland A's and deciding, as the sun came up, to all get hair weaves. One of the players kept his until the World Series, thus becoming the first player ever to come to bat in the Fall Classic wearing a toupee . . . Oh well, you get the idea.

So I invite all of you to come on in, the water's fine. So's the scotch or the bourbon or the vodka or the gin. And take it from someone who has gone through more glassware than Moe Greene in The Godfather: The bar patron's life is a fun life.

From *P.O.V.* Magazine, August 1997, pp. 57–61.

Diana Paxson is one of the leading fantasy writers of our time. This song is a homage to some of the great writers who inspired her. In particular, it was written to honor the Inklings, since it was her love for the work of Tolkien, Lewis, Williams, et al. which introduced her to science fiction fandom and the Mythopoeic Society, for which this song has become a tradition.

The Baby and the Bird

Diana L. Paxson

Old Rome had many taverns
Devoted to the vine,
Where Ovid pledged each new love
In red Falernian wine;
Catullus, shamed by Lesbia,
Poured out his grief in verse;
Apuleus noted follies,
And pondered which was worse.

Refrain:
But the place that draws me ever
When my fancy's running wild,
Is a little pub in Oxford
Called The Eagle and the Child,
The Eagle and the Child, oh,
Or else, as I have heard
Its regulars all called it—
The Baby and the Bird!

The company was lively
In Southwark's Tabard Inn,
When Chaucer and the Pilgrims

Were telling tales within,
And on the Canterbury road
They took that April day,
And at the other hostels
Where they stayed upon their way.

(REFRAIN)

When Villon, gutter-poet,
Reeled through the Paris night,
Drunk on verse and hypocras
And looking for a fight,
The Pomme de Pin, the Cheval Blanc
All welcomed him, and more,
With wine at every table
And doxies at each door.

(REFRAIN)

Of all the City's taverns,
When Bess was England's Queen,
The Mermaid, undisputed, ruled
The literary scene.
Each Global play was played again
And christened in brown ale,
When Shakespeare, or Ben Jonson,
Stood up to tell the tale.

(REFRAIN)

Augustan wits made merry
At London's Cheshire Cheese—
The topic was no matter,
So that the manner please—
Be it Love or Politicks,
'Twas scandalous, I've heard,
And Johnson had his Boswell
To write down every word.

(REFRAIN) Asking,

They sing of famous taverns,
But considering them all,
The one where I had rather
Been a fly upon the wall,
Would be the Inn where Tolkien,
Lewis, Williams too,
Met with the other Inklings
Asking, "Who has something new?"

Another Sports writer, Loverro is as given to romantic fancy as any of the breed. Here we see him invoke one male icon in defense of another. Alas, as all too often happens, reality is doomed to triumph over fantasy.

Death of a Bar

Thom Loverro

I was drinking Rolling Rock beer and smoking a genuine Cuban cigar in a roomful of people drinking Rolling Rock beer and smoking genuine Cuban cigars.

Why must all good things come to an end?

The death of a good bar can be a haunting experience. In Columbia, Md., the ultimate planned community—one giant Bennigans, if you will—it ranks as a tragedy that you can never forget. The night that Lucky Ned Pepper's closed down, forced out of business by a group of development weasels seeking to build a golf course community, was a night to mourn.

Yet it was also a night to celebrate—both sad and exhilarating, and I found the need to take a break from the wake. So I walked outside with my Rolling Rock beer and genuine Cuban cigar and sat on top of a picnic table away from the bar to reflect.

It has been said that if you eat the worm at the bottom of a bottle of Mexican mescal, you will have a vision. That's a pretty safe bet, since if you drink a bottle of mescal, you could eat Good Humor bars afterwards and still have visions.

I have never heard any such claims about the combination of Rolling Rock beer and genuine Cuban cigars.

Nonetheless, a figure began to materialize in front of me, and when I saw who it was, I thought that we could still save Lucky Ned Pepper's.

It was him. The Duke. John Wayne.

"Duke, Duke, you got here just in the nick of time. Can I call you Duke?" I asked him.

"That would suit me just fine, mister," the Duke said.

The Duke looked over at the bar and said, "When they fiesta in this town, they really fiesta."

175

"Yeah, but the party's over soon, Duke. Do you know what this bar is called? Lucky Ned Pepper's, after the gang that you shot up in 'True Grit,' " I said.

"Is Ned holed up in there?" he asked, reaching for his gun.

"No, no, Duke, the place is called Lucky Ned Pepper's, but it's really in honor of you. There's a large portrait of you hanging over the bar inside," I said.

"You've been trying real hard not to tell me something, Billy," the Duke replied, frowning.

"First of all, Duke, my name's not Billy," I said. "You see, there's a bunch of varmints in town that want to close Ned's down. And you're the bar's patron saint. You must have been sent here to stop them."

"That would cause me great annoyance and displeasure," he said.

"So how are we going to stop them?" I asked him.

The Duke looked over the land and said, "I'll need food for a week, water for 10 days, three pack horses and a good mule."

"What are you talking about, Duke? We're talking about a group of real estate weenies here, you don't need all that. Besides, we don't have 10 days. Are you OK? Do you want me to get you something to drink?" I asked him.

"You know, I can sleep cold, eat raw meat and raw fish, but come evening I sure miss my hot coffee," the Duke said, smiling.

"Fine, Duke, I'll see about getting you some raw meat and hot coffee later, but we don't have much time," I said. "We've got to stop these guys."

"Waiting is good for them and bad for us. It makes us careless, maybe dead," he said.

"That's right, Duke, we can't wait, so what's our next step?" I asked him.

"Well, I've seen unfriendly towns before. I know how to handle that," he said. "Could you tell me which one is the orneriest in the outfit?"

"I don't know, Duke. Couldn't you just appear before a couple of these developers and tell them that you wouldn't take too kindly to them shutting down Ned's?" I asked.

But then the Duke began to stammer. He reached back into his pocket and pulled out a rumpled old movie script.

"Well, they say the elk in Montana are as big as buffalo this year," he read from it. "We ought to go hunt 'em when this is all over."

It was then I realized that this vision of the Duke was the same one I had seen so many times on television, and all he could say were the lines from his films. So all I had to do was to get him on the right film script and maybe he could save Ned's.

But they didn't make John Wayne movies about town houses and golf courses and planned communities.

The Duke began to fade away. "How long does it take a man to ride to Pecos?" were his last words before the vision disappeared.

"Oh, I don't know, Duke, about three days if you take the interstates," I said sadly, to no one in particular.

The fiesta in the bar continued behind me as I tossed my cigar away and finished my beer. It was clear to me after that. There was no true grit in this town anymore.

 To drink is a pleasure, but at the Dresden it's an exception.
—CARL FERRARO, OWNER, THE DRESDEN ROOM, 1760 N. VERMONT AVENUE, HOLLYWOOD, CALIFORNIA

Life at Britain's Oxford University has traditionally been marinated in booze, as recorded in innumerable writings over the past two centuries. Despite the many changes suffered by the institution since the '60s, the following selection by a current undergrad shows that Oxford's alcoholic traditions remain alive and very well. For the uninitiated, a short Oxford glossary follows.

Alcohol—The Soul of Oxford

Edward Davies

At times, the Oxford Undergraduate of the 21st century begins to wonder whether the arrival of the bath was any compensation for permission to speak English rather than Latin at Formal Hall. Perhaps his tutors were right, before the advent of the undergraduette, to consider washing an unnecessary luxury for an eight-week term. He may, however, console himself with the thought that in the alcoholic field he clearly resembles those who came before him. His faithful tutor will still provide champagne to cure his colds, sherry to overcome his nervousness, and (for those who will not drink) "non-alcoholic" white wine. His sensitive disposition will still be disturbed by waking in evening dress at tea-time. His state of mind will be affected by the foolish College corkscrew. His Scout will still drink his Madeira. Hereafter the men in sherry-stained tweed may well consider themselves blessed, that they should have lived in the days of velvet-coated arm chairs and many holed tea strainers.

The tradition of "sconcing" at Formal Hall enables one undergraduate to challenge another (upon a point of honor) to drink without pause a yard of wine or ale. Those best acquainted with Hall Wine lean towards ale, although sconcing is more frequently attempted than carried out. A man who dares to set a pint glass of beer upon the table may reasonably expect not to be required to drink a larger glass of beer in expiation of his fault. For a request must be written in flawless Latin and passed up to High Table via a Servitor. It is then examined critically by the presiding Fellow. He is often mindful that the drink may be spilled over the clothes and gown not only of the sconced one, but those seated near to him. If there is anything which an Oxford don objects to, more than other Oxford dons, it is the horrid sacrilege of those who waste their drink. This is indeed a practice so abhorrent to him that he would rather stretch his sock across the table and balance a gilt-edged napkin on his nose, than allow undergraduates to set fire to a single mouthful of Chartreuse. Such parsimony leads High Table to prefer 1955 Port to a roof that does not leak. It means that undergraduates are traditionally given complimentary wine only on the Sovereign's Golden Jubilee. Which is to say, once every three hundred and fifty years.

Nevertheless, the personal generosity of the don is not to be doubted. It may surprise the unworldly reader to learn that very commonly (once a week, or thereabouts) we in this place are obliged to drink sherry from Portuguese bathroom glasses by men in gowns of green-tinged russel cord. This is called a tutorial, for those fortunate enough to study the Arts. A Fellow of Mathematics will never provide the fortified wine which is the source of all inspiration in the lives of Classicists or Historians. He is more likely to teach inverse multiplication by turning his student upside down and telling him to multiply.

But far be it that the reader should suppose the men of science men of restraint once they have put away their test tubes. This is no place to wonder in whose room the Cardinal Pole Society, one of Oxford's numerous clubs, left their Chaplain. We think not in which college's quadrangle the men of the Bullingdon, the Gridiron or the Canning last made merry. Nor may we inquire of the Dilettante Dining Club whether a solitary pineapple is capable of making a cocktail of a punch-bowl filled with gin. For most men, it is enough to hear the strangled cries of those members of Oxford drinking societies foolish enough to trespass on lawns sacred to the memory of aged porters.

In order to understand the true meaning of this strangled cry we must realize that the Oxford Porter has a weakness for wine glasses brimming with whisky. He can then happily be persuaded that he lives in the days when an undergraduate might be fined two-pence for chopping the Steward's toes off. But should so much as one toe be set upon the hallowed turf that is the Fellow's Lawn . . . It is wise indeed for the senseless undergraduate to recall that he who is thrown into Mercury Fountain is fined, not those who throw him in. The finest malt whisky that Oxford's wine merchants can provide will not save him now.

The undergraduate would do well also to remember the most important requirement of those sitting University Examinations. It is not the white bow-tie, suit, gown or mortar board. It is not the pink or white or red carnation (depending on whether it is the first or second or final examination). No, what matters most is that the ancient statutes of this happy institution provide that during his examination every undergraduate shall have a yard of his favored drink. How heroic these men are, that when they have sat for thirty-six hours of six days, they then consume a bottle of champagne before reaching their College. Again, so keen are the dons that not one drop shall be wasted, that, to monitor the Examination School crowds, they employ University Police. Their task is the proper removal of the champagne cork from the bottle. Their chief pleasure in this life derives from sawing the legs from the chair which, one recalls, once held the weight of the boy who was too fat. They are known for reasons apparent to any who have seen them, as 'the Bulldogs.'

Oxford drinking traditions are rarely intentionally begun. Indeed the most recent is the game of one-handed croquet now customarily allowed on the Feast of Candlemas by the Provost of Oriel College. The other hand is not absent, but merely otherwise employed in the consumption of Pimms-and-lemonade. This is more difficult than it appears when it must be made after six of the Senior Common Room's wines have been sampled in good measure.

This might perhaps alarm those who place their trust in the good sense of gilded youth, if the prose of this author has not sufficiently alarmed them already. But each year, at the moment when, by Act of Parliament, the hands of English clocks are sent back one hour, the rebellious undergraduates of Merton College walk backwards, anti-clockwise, around their quadrangle, deliberately drinking Merton College Port. They thus attempt to slow time down. Theirs is a noble attempt to recapture those precious five minutes of which every undergraduate in an essay crisis considers himself unjustly deprived by the arrival of the railways. How noble this is only those who have tasted Merton College Port will ever know.

Of course, nobody would ever consider writing a Collection Paper on Homer without the company of a bottle of Cognac. But the Oxford Undergraduate finds it too easy to sacrifice sensibility on the altar of drink. Who indeed would credit the well-washed young gentleman, who the day before produced a striking new interpretation of Kant's *Groundwork for the Metaphysics of Morals* with these words: "Today I met a young lad, walking up the gravel path towards the library in third quad. I asked him the way to the club. And he began to twitch, and when I asked him again, he played with the tie he was wearing: yellow it was, with purple spots. And when I pointed out that if it was necessary, I could produce a small vehicle, he ran back up the winding path until he had become a small tweed rectangle in the middle-distance. And I went and hid in a bush."

Who would deny that this man, so well acquainted with every age except his own, has been prepared for the real world, in which he will fulfil his rightful destiny as Member of Parliament, Judge, General or Bishop? Who else could quaff the dregs of the star-studded goblet, leap the fence of the college, swim the river at night and write all alone his essay? One man, or so each man thinks. And the dons look askance with a smile.

GLOSSARY OF TERMS (IN NO PARTICULAR ORDER)

Undergraduette: Female undergraduate.

Porter: bowler-hatted Guardian of the Gate at Oxford and Cambridge colleges, renowned in song and story.

Don/Tutor/Fellow: An amenable, elderly gentleman entrusted with the education of English youth; denied the right to birch undergraduates thirty years ago.

High Table & Senior Common Room: A number of dons, respectively eating or reposing.

Collection Paper: In theory, a silent, supervised College Examination. In practice, the institutionalization of plagiarism; a Latin scrawl written in undergraduate rooms.

Scout: the maid or manservant with which every Oxford undergraduate is entrusted; traditionally the most obliging man in Europe.

Servitor: Waiter at Formal Hall; originally one of the poorer undergraduates.

Formal Hall: Dinner in suit and gown preceded by Latin college grace

 Once found, and having supped at the Mitre, it is an experience
never to be forgotten.
—DON O'SULLIVAN, LANDLORD YE OLDE MITRE, 1 ELY COURT, ELY PLACE, LONDON, ENGLAND

From contemporary Oxford we travel back to contemporary New York, where a play-wright and essayist surveys the part alcohol plays in modern metropolitan life and love.

The Uses and Abuses of Alcohol

Jonathan Leaf

When the dress designer Oleg Cassini asked the Latin Diplomat and lothario Porfirio Rubirosa how it was that women so often went to bed with him, Rubirosa looked at Cassini a moment and then asked him if he had ever heard the expression, "I got her drunk and f—ed her."

Cassini said he had.

Rubirosa shrugged and then said, "That's it."

I suspect there is a lesson here.

No wise man drinks straight booze for the taste. Gin smells like bicarbonate—but with a drier after-taste. Whiskey makes your eyes water. Grappa hits your tongue like battery acid. Rum is vomited two ways: on your own and after you've been struck by the sort of people who are serious about drinking it. And vodka barely has a flavor.

During the enlightenment people in Europe drank wine and beer because the ground water was unsafe, as most rivers were infected by cholera and polluted with human excrement. Wine and beer in those days were very low alcohol concoctions and what fermentation there was in these beverages served to disinfect them. Beer and wine did not dehydrate. They were the main way by which people got water safely into their veins in an age when Europeans typically extracted iron from meteorites, then using the metal for weapons of war rather than the material in cooking pots. (And without cooking pots, of course, there was nothing to be used for boiling and thereby purifying the infected ground water.) So, when a man drank and said there's "health," he was not being metaphorical, and it's unlikely a term like "salud" would have come into common usage had Renaissance Venetians had good water coming out of pipes in their homes.

Drink was literally a life-saver in those days.

Yet, even in North America, where fresh running water was plentiful, consumption was impressive. The Puritans were huge drinkers. On average they drank about three times as much as present-day Americans do.

To be fair these Puritans were a lot wilder than most Americans of today would guess: the age of consent in the Massachusetts Bay Colony was ten, half of all female newlyweds were pregnant and the average age of first marriage was fifteen. But still . . . let's be honest. Would the Puritans have drunk so much if they'd had much to do? The Puritans closed the theaters and the Opera Houses in London, outlawed bear-baiting and generally made it hard to do anything except go to their boring, rationalist Church services which were full of syllogistic arguments for God's existence and of a length that one might wish to meet him soon.

There have, of course, been great drinkers who were also great thinkers and great men of the world, folk living life to the fullest as they drank to the fullest. Foremost among these men surely was Winston Churchill, savior of the free world and nemesis of that teetotaling, vegetarian Hitler. Churchill, we know, enjoyed brandy and cognac. As the latter is a concentrated essence of the Champagne grape, we can see that he was determined to get the distilled essence of celebration.

And undeniably this is an admirable approach to life when you think hordes of Nazis may be headed straight for Dover, holding lists which place your name at the top.

It is good that Churchill could wind up wearing a lamp-shade, and even better that he stopped Hitler from turning more people into them. But it does stand to reason that he was more the exception than the rule. Would all that many people really wish to consume vast quantities of a known central nervous system depressant if they were already high on life?

This is not to say that liquor doesn't have its place. It does. Many Europeans think that their recent intervals of fascism and communism are much less strange than our attempt at Prohibition. I for one think this indicates that they may still be drinking too much, but doubtless we must look to their wisdom as they are a wise and industrious group who in recent years have raised the world's cultural level with important contributions like Jacques Tati, the Euro, and the Russian mafia.

I like sweet, girly drinks like Whiskey Sours, Frozen Strawberry Daquiris and, yes, even Pina Coladas. One of the few things I share with Dick Nixon is mutual affection for Trader Vic's. I think a man who knows who he is and is sure of his sexuality has nothing to be afraid of in admitting a taste for the low and boorish class of drinks.

And I know that I am not alone in these tastes. There are many shy, neurotic and solitary women whose love lives would be non-existent were it not for these potent and sugary concoctions.

The question is how I can meet them.

One part of the United States preserved from Puritanism is southern Louisiana; a place where drinking is as acceptable and public as breathing. Here, a native of the place describes a particularly delicious sort of home brew.

A Jolt of Drunken Joe

C. E. Richard

In colonial New Orleans, one item alone accounted for fully one-third of all imports to the city: Alcoholic Beverages.

Furthermore, in a comparative study of other cities from the same period (Boston, Philadelphia, New York), New Orleans easily outmatched all North American towns in the ratio of pubs-to-per-capita-population. There was a tavern on virtually every corner of the French Quarter (and this remains true today, of course). This not only scandalized the Americans who visited the city, but they were also appalled to see blacks and whites drinking together freely at the same bars. Drinking blurs not only the eyes, it would seem, but also the boundaries of race and class.

A few years ago when I was still teaching in New Orleans, I invited a few colleagues from the university over for a dinner party to celebrate the start of summer vacation. The weather was warm, so instead of coffee after the meal, I broke out a bottle of my own home-brewed coffee liqueur and served it with cream. Sweet and strong, it was more like a dessert than a drink.

One of my friends had brought as his date a nervous young grad student from the economics department. She was pretty, but painfully prim and, I think, a little intimidated by the intellectual bombast blowing across the table from some of my guests. So while the others ranted theory, the poor girl sat sipping her liqueur and doing her best to give a damn. The evening dragged on like this until, finally, I managed to steer the discussion her way and coax an opinion from her. Everyone waited. She tipped back her glass and emptied it, pursed her lips and narrowed her eyes as if weighing her words carefully, then drawled, "Ya'll, I'm so drunk!"

I had no idea until later how many of those tiny little glasses she'd knocked back while everyone else blathered, but clearly she liked my coffee. A lot.

She held out her glass for me to refill. "Yummy!" she cooed and grinned at me. And that was the extent of her elocution for the rest of the evening.

If you've ever been blindsided by a good liqueur, then you know already what those sweet, sucker-punching drinks can do. And perhaps more than any other, a coffee cordial is pure guile. Its flavors seduce the palate of the unwary, tempt you to think that such a tasty little libation must be harmless. (Hey, it's served with milk. Milk's good for you, right?) Then it knocks you on your java-drinking ass.

But if you check your consumption, a coffee liqueur is an ideal after dinner drink, especially in the summertime. Served with a little chilled cream, it's cool, invigorating, and deliciously sweet. It also tends to engender a feeling in the drinker unlike other liqueurs. On the one hand, the alcohol has a calming effect, but the caffeine sharpens your senses just a bit and keeps you from slipping into that drowsiness that settles in after a good meal. Relaxed, but mentally alert—an ideal state of mind in a social setting.

Kahluha is easily the most popular coffee liqueur on the market. But at $40 for the large bottle, the notion of brewing your own becomes attractive—especially once you realize how quick and easy it is. And, whether serving it to guests or bringing it as a hospitality gift to someone else's dinner party, the uniqueness of a home-brewed liqueur never fails to win the appreciation of others.

That is, if it tastes good.

Coffee liqueur consists of nothing more than coffee, alcohol (usually vodka), sugar, and vanilla. It's a very simple recipe. But to make a good coffee liqueur, you have to begin by brewing a good pot of coffee. And there's a lot more to that than just plugging in the percolator.

"If you're going to the trouble of brewing your own liqueur, you obviously care about how it tastes. That means you have to start with the best ingredients available," says Clarke Cadzow, proprietor of Highland Coffees, among the very first gourmet coffee houses to open in South Louisiana.

Clarke is so painstaking in his devotion to quality coffee that he makes Juan Valdez look like an indifferent bean-picker. To many folks in Baton Rouge, Clarke Cadzow is Mr. Coffee. He knows just about everything that goes into a good cup of joe, and he's always ready to tell you about it.

"Coffee has a surprisingly large number of chemical compounds. It's a very complex substance," Clarke explains, citing studies by chemists who quantify flavor.

"Physiologically, human beings like the stimulation of all those different compounds. You may not realize it consciously, but chemically there's so much happening in your mouth when you drink coffee, and that's part of what we perceive as the pleasure of drinking it."

Take that, Mrs. Olsen.

There are lots of recipes for coffee liqueurs available on the Internet and in print but, inexplicably, they all seem to call for the use of instant coffee. So what's wrong with instant coffee, you ask? Well, let's just say that if the best part of waking up is Folgers in your cup, then I would advise you to crawl back into bed and curse the dawn. And if you hope to brew the kind of cordials that make grad student girls giggle and coo at your dinner parties, then keep in mind Clarke Cadzow's recommendations:

❏ Get freshly roasted coffee. "Coffee that isn't freshly roasted has only a shadow of the flavor it should," says Clarke.

❏ Use a manual drip pot, not an automatic or a percolator. A manual drip allows you greater control over the process. Not only does it make a better pot of coffee, but a manual drip is cheaper than an automatic.

❏ The liqueur demands a strong, concentrated coffee, so use a ratio of 4 tablespoons of coffee to every 6 oz. of water. Also, finer grounds (such as a large espresso grind) will brew stronger.

❏ Use pure water. If you take it from the tap, use cold water; hot water sits in your water heater tank, picking up impurities that can affect taste.

❏ Don't use boiling water. The optimal water temperature for drawing the maximum flavor from the grounds is between 195–205 degrees.

❏ Choose a mellow, full-bodied bean, such as a Sumatran or Central American coffees. They're lower in acidity and make a smoother liqueur. As for the roast, opt for the Viennese (half dark roast, half medium).

RECIPE:

    4 cups brown sugar
    2 ½ cups strong coffee
    A fifth of quality vodka (80 proof)
    2 tablespoons of Melipone Mexican vanilla

Combine sugar and coffee in a saucepan and simmer, stirring until sugar dissolves. Allow to cool to room temperature, then add vodka and vanilla. Mix well. Serve with chilled cream, half-and-half, or whole milk.

For a stronger, sharper liqueur, add ten whole roasted coffee beans to the mixture and store in a dark place for three weeks. Strain and filter before serving.

Dinner at Musso and Frank's

Ken O'Steen

I pulled a week's worth of letters and advertisements from the box I kept in Toluca Lake. Once a week was about as often as I checked. I threw it all in the trash except for one of the letters. It had been sent by Caca magazine. I read it, standing in the post office door. My story had been accepted, it would appear in the issue after next. Payment would come in the form of copies. I took the letter back inside, and wrote on the bottom of it with the post office pen. I asked the magazine to send the payment copies to another address. They were to be delivered to me, care of my ex-wife, I wrote, then I printed out her home address. They would never reach me of course, since my whereabouts were not available to her. But they weren't intended for me, they were intended for her.

Five weeks later, at the Barnes and Noble in Burbank, the issue with my story was on the shelf. I mentioned it to no one as was my practice. Not that there was anybody in particular to tell. Except for my ally Guthridge, who knew only that I wrote, but not that I published, there were no confidantes to tell. But with the "ad hoc friends," the blur of acquaintances, the randomly encountered, randomly employed, and endlessly biz-infatuated Hollywoodians it was never mentioned. This was my preference; my own measure of what I was, and what I did . . . and why.

Sheri as usual I had told that I'd finished a story . . . though I'd left it at that. Nevertheless she said, "We should celebrate." She invited me to something she called, "a gathering," at Musso and Frank's in Hollywood. It would be a "working party" for her she said. The hosts of the party were her roommate Darla's "clientele." All she knew Sheri said was that "they're in the business."

The two of them picked me up. On the way Darla congratulated me for "finishing that story," and guaranteed that everything all evening would be "on the tab." Sheri whispered to me, "Cept you'll probably have to find another way home, ok?"

Twelve or thirteen people occupied two tables pushed together in the back room. Most of them were men, a few were women, which surely explained the presence of Sheri and Darla. I was assigned a seat between one of the men and one of the women. The man next to me, in his conversation with the rest, alluded six or seven times in the initial fifteen minutes I was there, to the fact that he had directed a film. When the time came I ordered a drink and a steak. For the most part I kept my mouth shut. The men didn't notice much of anything except for Sheri and Darla; and perhaps two of the remaining four women who were attractive. The blonde next to me confessed forthrightly that she was a producer. I elicited the information by asking her what she did, though only after she'd asked me the question first. I had answered, "I ask for change due to the fact I'm homeless." She laughed, thinking no doubt that I was wry.

At some point, noticing a man standing at the bar, I nudged the fellow beside me and told him, "That guy looks like George Stephanopoulos." My tablemate looked at me blank-faced. "I know it isn't him, but he looks exactly like him, don't you think?"

"I've heard the name. Who is he? I can't recall."

"George Stephanopoulos, the presidential advisor? Left the job not long ago?"

"The name is familiar."

"Well he looks just like him."

"Right."

The next time I spoke to the man was when somebody made a reference to Marilyn Monroe. I nudged the man and said, "I wonder if Seymour Hersh had that fact in his book?" It was a little sarcasm, aimed at the dubious veracity of the salacious remark. "The Dark Side of Camelot," the book about JFK had just come out, and was everywhere in the news.

"Who?"

"What?"

"Who is that?"

"Seymour Hersh or Marilyn Monroe?"

"Marilyn Monroe." His face was twisted.

"Sorry . . . but . . . Seymour Hersh, the journalist? Wrote the books about My Lai, Kissinger . . . the KAL downing?"

"Oh."

The dinner was finished, and everyone was draining their drinks and ordering more. The blonde next to me was entirely attentive to the man on her other side. The words "residuals" and "scale" were overheard more than a few times. I smiled at Sheri and she smiled back . . . then took a cherry from the bottom of her glass and put it to the lips of the man whose ardors she had drawn for the night. One of the men had Darla's hand gingerly working his lap, it was plain to see. I drank and stayed quiet, reminding myself that the drinks were free. When the man beside me asked if I had seen *Titanic,* after someone else had brought the subject up . . . and he had realized he had nothing else to do momentarily but stare silently at his drink, I answered, "no, I haven't seen any movies at all for a while."

"See it. You really should."

"It's hard for me to believe it could top 'A Night to Remember,' except in special effects."

"I haven't seen that. It was about the Titanic?"

"Yeah."

"When was that?"

"Long time ago . . . it was in black and white."

"Hmmm."

"Course I would still like to see the ship sink . . . in the 200 million dollar version."

"It's awesome. Very thrilling. Really amazing."

The waiter came by and gathered a round of orders. Whether he had forbearance in expectation of a huge tip, or had learned to ignore the after dinner manifestations of lust and booze, or whether he was simply diminished in his senses, he moved around the table neither indignant nor sharing the mirth, unflappable, even though the roiling concupiscence was right there in his face. Other diners in the room seemed a bit less stoic, if the glances I intercepted en route to the table were any indication. The man beside me and I were left to stare forlornly at each other. The others were better occupied. So I asked, knowing I would likely regret it, "I believe you mentioned that you're a director?"

"Yeah. I direct."

"What are you working on right at the moment?"

"Right now, I have an idea in development with my agent. It would be a theatrical film of the tv show *Bonanza.* In this, the Cartwrights will end up with a baby somehow. They'll be raising it . . . comedy, with some tender moments."

"Okay. I see." He spared me the need to elaborate.

"What did you say it is you do?"

"I didn't . . . but I'll tell you. I'm working right now on a script. A biopic of Camille Paglia."

"Camille Paglia, the actress?"

"A different one."

"Oh." When he turned his head I got up from the seat. I took my drink with me and moved to the bar. I ordered another martini and pointed back at the table. "Put it on our check, please." Rather than my usual vodka, I was drinking the famous Musso and Frank martinis, reputedly the best in town.

I had been seated at the bar ten minutes or so when a woman's voice behind me said, "Hello again." It was the blonde producer who had been sitting next to me at the table. She took the seat beside me at the bar. "Tired of talking business," she said, putting down her drink.

"I can see why," I said, and smiled.

"Everybody says the business is awful . . . and they all desperately want to be in it."

"I don't."

"Really. I thought I heard you mention something over there about a script."

"I was lying."

"Oh," she laughed. "So you should be in the business then." After the both of us laughed, she began to tell me about her present work . . . despite having told me just before that she was tired of talking about exactly that. Then she said, "You look to me like an actor."

"Please."

"What do you mean pulleeze?"

"I'm no actor. What I am is an unemployed poet. I went to the unemployment office just today; they didn't have a single job for a poet."

She laughed and said, "You aren't going to answer me are you?"

"I don't think so. I have worked. I've had jobs before."

"Thanks. Thanks for being completely forthcoming." In truth, she didn't seem to care at all. And besides, it was time to reload our drinks. She looked well on the way to getting completely plastered, if she wasn't already. The closer she got, the more risqué, the more suggestive her conversation became of course. She finally whispered, "So how do you feel about spanking?"

 Everyone "says" we make the best martinis in L.A.—you be the judge.
—MANNY AGUIRRE, BARTENDER, MUSSO AND FRANK'S 6667 HOLLYWOOD BOULEVARD, HOLLYWOOD, CALIFORNIA

From the unpublished novel, *Hills and Assassins*.

Yet another rare alcohol-friendly subculture in the United States is the "Holy Land" of Kentucky, an area that has given us that most American of drinks, Bourbon. Here, a report from the front.

My Old Kentucky Bourbon

Martin Booe

Kentucky, where I was born and raised, endured the Civil War as a so-called neutral state. The word "neutral" in this case is a fairly treacherous adjective. The fact is that the war tore Kentucky asunder, dispatching its sons in more or less equal portions to North and South, so there wasn't much neutral about it. But then Kentucky has always been of two minds about itself, and I can't help reflecting that it was precisely my state's very schizophrenic nature that dressed it as the stage upon which bourbon, our only indigenous American spirit, would first appear.

Consider, for example, that Kentucky ushered in modern Pentecostalism with the Cain Ridge Revival, in Bourbon County, in 1801. Consider too that it was also in Bourbon County, in the late 1700s, that a renegade Baptist minister named Elijah Craig invented the state's poison of choice, an apostasy from the doctrine of sobriety that, according to lore, saw him run out of several churches. (There is also of course tobacco, race horses, and more recently cannabis—Kentucky has long been a prodigious purveyor of vices—but let's stick with bourbon.) At any rate, bourbon and religion have been long viewed as opposing forces, but then, maybe they needed each other. (In Bourbon County itself, religion won; the precinct is today "dry," meaning the sale of alcohol is prohibited.)

Growing up Catholic, an anomaly in those parts, I was largely spared from this dualistic view of the spirit world, but not entirely. My maternal grandparents were Baptists, grandma a teetotaler and grandpa nearly so. On the rare occasion that my grandfather imbibed, it was, as they say, for medicinal purposes, at least in theory. He kept on hand a pint of a particularly rotgut brand whose name I can't remember. It was stored in back of the refrigerator, shrouded in its brown paper bag. He used to say that whiskey should have a "bite" to it, and I would imagine this one bit hard. After all, it was medicine, and medicine isn't supposed to taste good.

It is probably no coincidence that a good number of Kentucky's distilleries are situated in and around Bardstown in Nelson County, a sandbar of staunch Catholicism jutting up amid a sea of Baptists, and therefore a good deal friendlier to whiskey. This is where my father's side of the family hailed from, and here bourbon was regarded as something almost sacramental. The material world being corrupt, bourbon offered a much-needed transport to the realm of the spirit, literally and figuratively. This was acknowledged as one's due. Though excess was far from unknown, it wasn't the rule. For the more settled ones, this means of passage was a gondola, gently ferrying them to quieter realms; for the wilder it was a rocket launcher, catapulting them into the giddy stratosphere.

Those of the clan who stayed on the farm worked at the distilleries during the winter months. As a rawboned young buck, my Uncle Frank, upon taking leave of the house of a Saturday night, pint of Jim Beam in the breast pocket of his overalls, would invariably be accosted by my grandmother, who'd inveigh him: "Frank! Don't forget your rosary!" Thus, religion and bourbon rarely parted company, although I doubt that Uncle Frank racked up a single novena down at what my mom always referred to as the Ave Maria Beer Joint. (It was a coinage inspired by the statue of the virgin mounted over the doorway of the small roadhouse where they congregated.) When I was a child and visiting my grandmother at the farm, Frank would stomp into the kitchen and in what seemed like a spontaneous outburst of goodwill, offer to take my brother and me for a ride in his pickup. Years later, my mom told me we were his cover for running bootleg whiskey to so me of the neighboring dry counties. "Just takin' the boys for a ride, officer!"

Kentucky's early distillers—moonshiners—were, almost to the last strand of DNA, some combination of Scottish, Irish and English, and their making of whiskey ("whisky in the old world") was, in a way, strangely Calvinistic, an homage to self-reliance and an assertion of individual rights. But in Kentucky, even in the Catholic part of the state, even despite the perhaps withering but still discernible Celtic roots, the bottle is never placed center table as it is in Scotland and Ireland. The drinking was hardly surreptitious, but there was a certain wariness about public consumption that kept the bottles to the side. Still, it was part of the culture.

My grandmother died when I was fourteen, and after her funeral, I was astonished (and delighted) to have a beer thrust into my hands at her wake. The party soon dissolved into a warm bath of familial geniality, horseshoe games and for the younger, mumblypeg. More to the point, and largely thanks to bourbon, it dissolved into tribal mourning and in this was much joy. It was a far cry from the starchy funeral receptions typical of my native Frankfort, only 60 miles away, but a much stiffer place.

My father had died when I was an infant; when I was five, my mother remarried, to a man who became my real father. He had moved back to Kentucky after 13 years on the east coast to take over the candy business his mother had started. Its piece de resistance was bourbon candy, which his mother had invented, probably in a fit of whimsy, and it had caught on. (His mother's mother was an English Catholic expatriated to Kentucky, hence the relatively libertine attitude toward drink.) She started Rebecca-Ruth Candies in 1919, with her friend, Rebecca Gooch—hence the folksy if unimaginative name. The business had nursed them through the lean years of the depression.

Their first success was the Kentucky Mint Colonel, a mint cream covered in dark chocolate and topped with a salted pecan. At some point shortly after the repeal of prohibition, a friend mentioned that his two favorite tastes were a sip of bourbon and a bite of one of "Miss Ruth's" Kentucky Colonels. Inspiration struck. The idea of chocolate and bourbon together conjured unimaginable delights. Miss Ruth spent two years perfecting her recipe, and while I can't say with total certainty that she was the first person to hit on the combination, there's nobody around to argue to the contrary. At any rate, the bourbon ball gradually became a regional favorite.

It is one thing to be a kid whose dad owns a candy factory, and quite another thing when the candy features bourbon as its most notable ingredient. As it happened, this served me well.

I was an electro-magnet for bullies. I didn't know how to fight and worse, I LOOKED like I didn't know how to fight. Unfortunately, the walk home from school led past Second Street Elementary, highly regarded as a training institute for the most talented of local junior toughs, who naturally regarded us parochial school kids, in our white shirts and clip-on neckties, as easy quarry.

About a week into first grade, I was set upon by a hulking specimen of boyhood nicknamed Lurch. He gave me a bloody nose, an experience he found sufficiently gratifying to bear repetition. Soon Lurch awaited me daily at the end of the St. Clair Street Bridge. I knew I couldn't out-tough Lurch, but I had a secret weapon. The next time I met up with him, I reached into my pocket and pulled out a fistfull of bourbon balls. Violence . . . or chocolate? For Lurch, the choice was easy. Soon he became not merely my friend but my defender as well, and when problems with other bullies arose, all I had to do was conjure his name and the trouble would vanish.

My encounter with Lurch would not be the first time I would use candy to mollify my tormentors. Nobody dislikes being given chocolates, but in my experience bourbon candy has a singular power to make women swoon and to diffuse aggression in Type-A personalities. I believe they have saved me from being fired more than once; proffering bourbon balls as gifts, I have appeased several bosses who clearly suffered from borderline personality disorder. It's not the booze, really. Although they carry a bit of a punch, you can't blame their mood-altering effects on the alcohol; you'd put yourself in a diabetic coma long before you could eat enough of them to blow 0.8 on a breathalizer.

These days, I feel fortunate to live in what amounts to a bourbon renaissance. The quality of bourbon suffered terribly after the repeal of prohibition. Faced with a sudden, unprecedented spike in demand, distilleries unjudiciously blended what little stock remained with unfinished swill, and the result was today's industrial-produced bourbon. The prevailing infatuation with single-malt scotch spurred the bourbon industry to follow suit. The proofs are higher and the quality is better. That is something to which we can all raise a glass.

In the years since I left home, I have traveled around the world to find that bourbon is alive and well. From India to Vienna, I find that my birthright affords me a peculiar status. "Kentucky! Bourbon!" And my host will pull out a dusty bottle of Jim Beam or more likely Jack Daniels, which technically is not bourbon (it's made in Tennessee and is therefore denied the moniker). Whatever the label, there's a fifty percent chance that it was made in my home town, in which case I am greeted like a conquering king.

From Kentucky we return to Southern California; but the Bourbon will follow us into consideration of an unsophisticated drink that nevertheless still packs a punch and commands a following.

The Boilermaker

Lou Matthews

A Boilermaker is an unmixed drink: It's a shot of bourbon or whiskey, chased with a beer. Your stomach does the mixing, and something more, I think. Cold fusion or an hallucinogenic reaction, some small rebellion. You sip the bourbon, swallow the beer and then it kicks back, a slow punt lofted up the neural sheath. You feel it at the base of your skull and think about hang-time as it travels, pleasurably, up to that small patch inside your pate where spine shivers start.

I don't drink Boilermakers often. My usual evening drink is bourbon with a splash of water. On hot days I like beer. When I drink beer I get a comfortable lazy feeling. Bourbon keeps me alert. Bourbon makes me think that I'm thinking.

Boilermakers are a wild man's drink. None of the usual sobriety sensors work with Boilermakers. With Boilermakers, you are suddenly over that edge, slurring, without a clue that you were close.

I know I'm over that edge when I start eating everything in sight. It's a matter of ballast. Trying for balance. I really don't like to be drunk; I like that nice loose imaginative stage this side of drunk and I eat, when I drink, to stay on this side. With Boilermakers, though, food doesn't really help. I don't slow down. Even while I'm eating, I keep setting up that shot and a beer.

On the night that I'm thinking of, I'd gone back to Maddy's house. Maddy is my friend Madden. Madden Davis. Maddy wasn't there but I have a key; he decided, when I started teaching at the university, that I should have a place to hole up. He's a good friend, Maddy, he knows how small a town Loma Linda can be.

I'd just finished office hours—nine hours to talk with fifteen students, and look at their new work. Most of them were doing watercolors. There was some catching up to do. I was making up two weeks of cancelled office hours.

My mother had been in the hospital. The tumor was malignant. It was confined, they hoped, to the uterine area. She would have radiation therapy, to shrink the tumor and slow the cancer. The doctors wanted to do a hysterectomy after that.

At Maddy's there was beer in the refrigerator, Mickey's Big Mouths. It's a barrel-shaped bottle with a big mouth. After nine hours of talking, I was dry enough to inhale one. The first sip was amazing. Cold, almost sweet, it was a slap at the back of my head and a long descending shudder. I finished it and opened another.

It was just six. There would be another hour of light. I finished half the second beer and, thirst and dry throat gone, wished it was bourbon. I wanted the clarity of bourbon.

I checked the liquor cabinet. There was a liter bottle of Jack Daniels on the bottom shelf, with about one good shot left. Maddy would have been disappointed. He prefers to anticipate his friends' needs. He takes friendship and hospitality most seriously.

Maddy comes from an old Virginia family and even though they ran out of the money about three generations ago, he still has their generous instincts. He just can't afford all of them all of the time. Maddy's other family inheritances are a wonderful soft accent and more manners than can be used in California.

I considered the whiskey. I wanted a jolt before I drove the freeway. The commute—Loma Linda to L.A.—is 80 miles. I've been driving both ways, twice a week, for three years, long enough to know every flicking building, light, sign and off-ramp, peripherally and by heart. Long enough to be dulled by the drive. The jolt is to change perception, to make myself more interesting, which makes the commute tolerable.

If Maddy had been home he would have rolled me a joint. I only smoke grass when commuting, to avoid tickets. Maddy decided it would be a good way to slow me down. When I got bored by the commute, I tried to shorten it by speeding up. I'd gotten two tickets, the last a charitable 80 in a 55. One more ticket and my insurance premium would double. Two, and my license would be lifted.

Maddy worked out the equation. Two hits and I drove comfortably at 60, eyes wide, a buzz in my head and the wire taut between my shoulder blades. The grass also provided the necessary paranoia. I drove with the constant sense that a Highway Patrolman was there, drafting along in my blind spot. Waiting for mistakes. Fear kept the wire taut and my foot light.

I poured the shot of whiskey into a short glass, adding a cube of ice. The whiskey tasted sharp, after the beer.

I sipped both. When the beer was gone there were still a few sips of whiskey so I opened another Mickey's. When the shot was done, there was still two thirds of a beer. I went back to the closet. In the back, behind the scotch, was a bottle of Old Fitzgerald. Old Fitzgerald sounds like one of those Thriftimart soundalike brands, but it is actually a fine whiskey. I poured a shot of Old Fitzgerald.

I was nearly through the second shot, pleased at the way it was all working out—the whiskey and beer levels now nearly equal and a dead heat in sight—when I found myself in the refrigerator, rummaging through the hydrators.

There was a heel of salami, a half-wedge of swiss cheese, half a pickle. There were Carr's water crackers in the cupboard. I took it all back to the table and started cutting things off and stacking them up.

It all tasted wonderful, that's another effect of Boilermakers. After the pickle was gone I went back and found a hardboiled egg and some green olives. I cut the egg in half and spooned on a little russian dressing. I popped olives like they were peanuts. There was still some salami and three crackers when the second Boilermaker was gone. I decided, shrewdly I thought, that I should break the beer cycle. I poured a whiskey and water to round everything off.

I believe that I cleared the dishes, I hope that I washed them. My main ambition, as I recall, was to get on the road while there was still light. It seemed important. It was about seven when I reeled out the door and stared up at the sky.

It was just light. The tops of the palm trees along Roscoe Avenue were distinct, hard-edged against the bright blue sky, but the lower trunks were shadowed. On smoggy days the twilight in Loma Linda is a golden haze. When there is wind, as there was that day, when it is clear, the air is nearly silver-colored in the gloaming.

I stood by the car with my hands stretched out flat on the roof. There was a light warm breeze coming down Roscoe, picking up the heat of the pavement and the scent of the orange blossoms. It was exactly seven. The sprinklers in Maddy's front lawn, which are on a timer, dribbled and gasped and spurted, then shot up steady circles of beads. The drops sprang out of shadow, reached their height, glistened there in the remaining band of sunlight, then dropped to the darkening grass.

I watched the light hairs on my arms moving. The air, the beer, the whiskey, the breeze, the twilight; they all had something to do with my contentment. My shoulders felt light. Oiled. The hair on my neck felt the air. Every hair was a sensor, every pore was a nostril.

There was the first taste of the shade in the breeze now, I watched the chill bumps come up on my forearms. Closure. It was easy to get in the car. The seats were warm and the red leather was fragrant.

From the unpublished novel, *The Moon Reaches Down to Me.*

Three of the archetypal experiences are: a) the drunken serviceman on leave in exotic locale; b) the pub crawl from hell; and c) the surreal, near hallucinogenic evening that never ends. In this true-life experience, all three genres deftly merge.

Phantom Bar Crawl

Andrew Dove

In the fall of 1988, I remember being assigned to a classified organization in South Korea. I had always wanted to go to that country and partake of its great sport, the drinking of So-Jou. When I arrived the country was just beginning to feel those razor cold winds coming down from Manchuria.

When soldiers arrive "in-country" they normally go to the US military compound at Yongson, which is a military base in the middle of the city of Seoul. Seoul is the capital of Korea, once known as the "land of the morning calm." Across the street from Yongson is the garment district known as E-Tah-Wan. E-Tah-Wan was to be the site of one of my greatest drinking bouts.

In-Country veterans had warned me about the powers of So-Jou. They cautioned me "never drink alone, never drink a lot of the beverage." Well, one chilled night after I'd been there awhile and had some time to myself, I decided to leave the safety of the compound, cross the street, have some dinner and who knows . . . perhaps find a little So-Jou.

I didn't have to go very far into E-Tah-Wan. The area has a high concentration of small tailor shops. Many of them have restaurants on the second floor. These are little mom and pop shops, which would never pass health inspection over here, but are a charm of old Seoul. I selected one and walked up a creaky narrow staircase to the restaurant. Actually it was about the size of a large living room with only a few tables and a smiling gold-toothed proprietor. I sat down, and ordered my favorite Korean delight, Bulgogi. As I waited I asked the waitress that came out of nowhere if they had any So-Jou. She sort of smiled and glanced over at the gold-toothed one for guidance. Both seemed to share a knowing moment as she faced back to me with a huge smile and a "ohh, yes . . . you like so-jou, you number one . . . I take care of you."

I sat quietly while the initial Kim-Shi and other pickled vegetable bowls appeared. The girl disappeared behind a green curtain. In a few moments she returned with a very small coke-like bottle and what appeared to be a glass thimble. She said, "You enjoy . . . GI . . . You number one." I filled the thimble with a clear cool substance. I took my first swig and screeched "ahhhhhh, it burns!" The waitress giggled and said "you OK number one . . . you try more." I began to wonder if this stuff was OK. I tried another swig . . . it too burned. The bottle still contained a great deal of substance. How could I return to Young-San defeated? I resolved to finish the liquid.

After a few more swigs, I realized the fluids were actually quite mild. In fact I now realized the whole So-Jou legend was just that—a legend. Finally I finished the bottle and I felt just fine. Oh perhaps a slight buzz, but no more that a couple of beers. In fact it was downright delicious. I looked up at the gold-toothed one that now was smiling from lobe to lobe and ordered another. He and the waitress giggled once more as I finished my dinner. The dinner itself had become far more delicious than I ever remembered Korean food to be.

Additional So-Jou was brought to me. I filled one thimble after another till it was all gone. It was so smooth—so tasty. Then I realized I couldn't taste. At this point began one of the strangest evenings I can recall, or not recall. By now the waitress and the gold-toothed one were laughing . . . about what not me nooo . . .

I arose to my feet in order to pay the bill. That was the last continuous memory I was to have. As I rose it all went blank. Next I was in a strange honky-tonk somewhere in Seoul. Here I was in a strange bar, music blaring and a bargirl dancing and gyrating in a go-go disco light set-up. I had no idea where I was. At this moment the bartender arrived and asked me in heavily accented English "you and yaw girly want more beer?" I glanced over to my left and there tucked under my arm was a beautiful Korean woman wearing a leather vest over what appeared to be nothing and tight jeans. I remember asking her who she was.

The two chilled beers arrived and in my woozy state I heard him demand 200 Won. I reached for my wallet . . . no money. Naturally I asked if he took American Express. He disappeared with my card, as I tried to recall who my "date" was. I sort of drifted in and out . . . next the bartender returned screaming "NO TAKE AMERCAN EXPRESS" I rose . . . at this another blackout.

In the next vignette, I'm in some kind of apartment. My "date" from earlier was screaming 20,000 WON . . . 20,000 WON . . . and now the vest was off . . . I yelled back "I don't know you" . . . BLACK OUT.

I was running running faster faster through back alleys. I was like the one armed man in the old fugitive stories. BLACK OUT.

Nothing tied these bizarre scenes together.

All I remember was waking up back in my quarters at Yong-Son, sicker than a living man should be. Was it a dream . . . ?

The clue came a month later with an American Express bill for $250 for my date. The good news was I'd never signed anything. It was real but not really.

Bars, as will be abundantly evident by now, are often substitute families. Sometimes, as the following story makes clear, one becomes a black sheep. The loss of position can be just as devastating.

One for the Road

Mark Alessio

After staring out of his apartment window for two straight hours, lost in thought, Sal had decided upon Tuesday. He had run all the days of the week through his mind, trying to pinpoint the "feel" of each, cataloguing all the particulars. It was funny how each one had its own character, like neighbors . . . seven individuals living in seven apartments on the same floor.

Tuesday won by a nose, though, and Sal didn't change his mind once he decided. He stood up, then, his knees and backside aching from hours spent in the hard wooden chair, walked over to the dresser, and looked at himself in the mirror. He had made his choice, and he had chosen Tuesday as the day on which to commit the greatest act of betrayal since the kiss of Judas.

That solitary brainstorming session had occurred just last Friday, a hundred years ago by his reckoning. Now, Tuesday was here, and the last four days had slid by on greased rails, blurred into a single unit, the way the letters l-m-n-o-p sounded when a kid sang the alphabet. Patience would be the hardest part. It wouldn't make sense to go to Mickey's before eleven, Tuesday or not. Someone would be there until midnight came and went. Someone would be hanging around, hunched on a stool, hands folded on the edge of the old bar like it was a church pew. God, he'd done it for half of his life.

At ten forty-five, Sal shut off the television, picked up his plate, gilded now with the remains of a perfunctory dinner of macaroni and cheese, dropped it into the sink, and poured himself a tall glass of water from the tap. Resting one hand on the cool porcelain rim, he braced himself and downed the entire glass without stopping for breath. He placed the glass next to the plate and stared at the small still-life for a moment. Then, he put on his overcoat, opened the top dresser-drawer and reached underneath a pile of clean undershirts. His hand came out holding a .38-caliber revolver. Sal held it out before him, twisting his hand to get a look at every angle. He dropped the gun into his overcoat pocket.

It was Tuesday night. It was time to head to Mickey's Place, just as he'd done almost every night for more years than he could count. Shutting the apartment door hard behind him, Sal walked over to the stairway and began a quick descent. As he was just about to hit the main landing, a sound from below brought him up short. He sneaked back up a half dozen steps and listened, holding his breath. But the first-floor hallway was already quiet again, so he edged down the rest of the stairs and darted for the front door. That was definitely the super's door he heard slam as he was going down the stairs. With the rent two weeks late . . . *again!* . . . the super was high up on Sal's list of "people to avoid like the plague." Unfortunately, this list was a long one, and the others on it, the ones who occupied more prominent places, weren't the type to stop at slipping delinquent notices under his door.

It was a twenty-minute walk from Sal's apartment building to Mickey's Place. This was never an absolute quantity, though. It varied with mood, weather, and circumstance. If Sal was feeling mellow, usually on the return trip, the twenty-minute walk became a half-hour stroll. When he was in a hurry to get to the bar after a rough day, it became a twelve-minute dash. Taxi-rides in the rain, or snowbound sidewalks, added more variables to the equation. Then again, tonight was Tuesday, the "dead" night. In happier times, Sal would have been on his way home from Mickey's around now. He rounded the corner and stopped to gaze down the street.

It was a typical downtown street. The buildings weren't particularly tall, and they had seen a few generations come and go. The storefronts were all covered by those loose, half-rusted gates that always clanked in the wind like nervous metallic skeletons. All the cars were still and dark, nestled against the curb in their spaces. *The city never sleeps?* thought Sal. Heck, here it rolls over and slumbers like a baby.

Mickey's Bar was located below street level, its front steps flanked by heavy iron fencing painted a shiny black. Sal walked down the familiar half-dozen concrete steps and pushed open the door, causing Mickey to turn around from the cash register. He was a big man, his broad, open face topped by thinning black hair greased back until it shone. He was wearing the usual white shirt and black bow tie. When he saw Sal, his face broke into a wide grin.

"Sal! What the hell brings you here at this hour?"

"Hey, Mickey." He tried to smile as he said it, but it was more grimace than grin.

"Are you okay, Sal? Come and sit down, will ya?"

"Yeah, sure." He had been standing at the end of the bar, just standing there like a mannequin. If he was going to do this, he'd have to loosen up. Hey, life was like that, right? People sometimes had to do things that were distasteful, sometimes downright ugly. No one could predict all the—He realized Mickey had been speaking to him.

". . . okay?"

"Huh? What was that?"

"You must've really had a rough day, Sal. I said, 'Can I pour you a beer?' "

"Sure, why not?" He'd have to nurse it. Keep a clear head.

Mickey set the beer down and looked at Sal for a few seconds. "You gettin' sick, Sal? You look a little pale. You wanna talk?" When Sal shook his head, Mickey shrugged, walked to the end of the bar, and began leafing through a stack of invoices.

Sal turned and tried, as nonchalantly as possible, to size up the place. There were four other patrons in the bar besides himself. Three stools down from him was a man he knew, an old-timer named Franz Varshaw. Once upon a time, Franz had been a legend in the city. Sixty years ago, he was its most popular and widely-read reporter. He was the news for so many memorable decades. These days, his mind wasn't screwed-down as well as it might have been, and the great news scoops of his past bled through into the present like an old paint job showing through a one-coat whitewash. To his shock, Sal noticed that Franz was weeping very silently, staring down at his drink all the while. The sight brought him up out of his own thoughts for a minute, and he signaled to Mickey, who dropped the invoices he'd been rifling through, shoved his pencil behind his ear, and walked the length of the bar over to Sal.

"Franz is crying. Is he alright?"

Mickey shot the old man an affectionate glance. "Yeah. He's been like that off and on all night."

"Do you know why?"

"I've tried to piece it together. The best I can come up with is, on his way here he saw the Goodyear blimp and thought it was the Hindenburg. He'll be okay. In fact, I'm gonna call a cab for him right now."

As Mickey reached for the phone beside the old National cash register, Sal smiled for the first time that night. Serendipity!! One down, and all because he'd asked a simple question about an old reporter's tears. That still left three other patrons, though. Two of them, a relaxed couple of indeterminate middle-age, were sitting in a booth just behind him, drinking gin and tonics. On the worn vinyl seats beside each one sat a monogrammed bowling-ball bag. In the last booth sat a man by himself, holding a beer in one hand and a cigarette in the other, his back to the door. The man's short, curly hair and the set of his shoulders seemed familiar. With a flash, Sal recognized him. The flash was accompanied by a grenade exploding in the pit of his stomach. It was Tom Martinez. *Officer* Tomas Martinez, to the man on the street.

I don't believe this! It was the closest thing to a frustrated groan Sal could come up with in his thoughts, without actually vocalizing it. It must have been at least two months since Sal had seen Martinez here at Mickey's Place, killing some time after work. Everyone assumed he'd been transferred, or *something*. This could change everything in a hurry.

As this interplay of potential cause and effect took center stage in Sal's head, the man from the first booth walked over to the bar, set two empty glasses down with a thud, and called Mickey.

"Bartender. Two more gin and tonics. And, remember, no religious drinks, if you get my drift." He chuckled then, as though he'd just invented the world's most devilish joke. The chuckle was echoed loudly and with gusto from the woman sitting at his table.

Mickey looked at the man uncomprehendingly, then flashed the same look on Sal. Despite the mental cockfight that had taken the place of normal thought in his head, Sal still found enough presence of mind to be intrigued by the man's challenge.

"Excuse me," asked Mickey, eyeing the customer warily, "did you say something about religious drinks?"

"Yeah, I did. I said, 'remember, no religious drinks.'" He gave Mickey and Sal another few seconds to solve the mystery, to pick up his gauntlet. Then, he burst out, "Religious drinks, get it? Drinks that aren't wholly water, get it? Drinks that aren't watered down, don't you see? Wholly water . . . holy water? You see?" He spelled out "holy" to make his point.

"Yeah, yeah, I get it," mumbled Mickey, as he made the drinks. He gave the customer his best professional smile, while keeping his finger an extra three seconds on the tonic pump. He took the man's twenty, made change, and slammed the cash register door shut. As he turned back, he saw that Sal had been looking at him, turning away quickly when their eyes met.

Sal sipped his beer slowly for a while, paging through a copy of yesterday's paper which had been left on the bar. He looked at the old Bulova clock hanging over the cash register. It was one of those timeless pieces—'Timeless pieces.' Hey, Mr. Bowling-Ball would choke on that. Clocks . . . 'timepieces' . . . 'timeless pieces' . . . Get it? Ha-ha!—that seemed designed to measure the nighttime hours, and only the nighttime hours. The minute and hour hands were black arrows that didn't just point to the hours; they stabbed them, pinned them hard to the old clock face, illumined gently by a weary, mild, buttermilk light. It was a little moon hanging there, ringed all around with numbers. The small moon said it was now 12:23. Tuesday had given way to Wednesday. Sal slipped his hand into his coat pocket and rested it against the revolver. Wasn't "cold metal" the standard description for guns, whether nestled in pockets or jabbed into backs? This gun felt warm, warm with his own body heat.

Finally, the couple at the table downed the last of their gin and tonics, sidled out of the booth and headed out the door. They walked up the concrete steps to street level, their arms entwined, their free hands carrying their bowling-ball bags. Sal watched their legs pass by the length of the window, then turned back at the sound of Mickey's angry voice on the phone.

"Gimme a break! Do you know how long his poor old guy's been waiting? He's gotta go home. No, I'm not calling you a liar. If you say you dispatched a car, then you dispatched a car. All I'm saying is, the guy's alone . . . well, of course he can wait for you to send another cab . . ."

"Hold it." It was Martinez who said that. Officer Martinez. He spoke so suddenly it made Sal jump. His hand was still resting against the warmth of the .38 in his coat pocket. From the corner of his eye, he saw Martinez leave his booth and head towards him. Wondering if anyone had seen him flinch, he slowly withdrew the hand from his pocket. He took a casual pull on his beer, turned to Martinez and said, "Hey, Tom! I thought that was you over there."

"Sal! Good to see you. Excuse me a second." He turned to Mickey, who was holding his hand over the mouthpiece of the receiver. "Listen, Mick, there's no reason Franz has to wait for a cab. I'll take him home. I was about ready to leave anyway." Sal smiled involuntarily. Serendipity . . . again?

"You sure, Tom?"

"Absolutely. Come on, old-timer, let's head home." He rested a hand on Franz's shoulder and gave it a friendly shake.

"Oh-h-h, the humanity," mumbled Franz, another tear rolling down his leathery cheek. "No, I'll stay. I want to forget."

Sal's chest tightened at the possibility of such a fortuitous turn of events getting mucked-up because of an old man's stubbornness. He had to think fast. "Franz," he began, almost instinctively. The aged reporter turned a weary face to him.

"You're never going to meet your deadline at this rate," he continued. Martinez and Mickey smiled at each other over Franz's bowed head.

"Deadline?"

"You'd better get some sleep, Franz. You've got a lot of work ahead of you. They'll be expecting copy as soon as you can punch it out. Since Tom is heading in your direction . . ." He knew he was acting in Franz's best interests, but he still felt lousy doing this to him.

"What do you say, Franz?" added Martinez. "Sal's got a point. Shall we get going?" Without another word, Franz slipped down slowly from his stool and shuffled towards the door. As Martinez turned to follow him, he grabbed Sal's arm. For one white-hot second, Sal's whole world was reduced to a gun in a pocket, an object of mass, one that would weigh the cloth of any overcoat down just enough . . . just enough for someone with experience in these things to pierce the disguise and see the sagging fabric for just what it was.

"Thanks, Sal. We'll talk next time, okay?" Martinez gave Sal's arm a squeeze and turned away to open the door for Franz.

When the two men had left the field of vision allowed by the bar's windows, Mickey set another beer down in front of Sal. "That was quick thinking. Cheers!"

"Cheers!" A buyback? The last thing Sal needed right now was a buyback, a token of affection from someone he was about to betray for a bag of silver. It was time. It was definitely time. Just then a question came to him so clearly, and with such a kick, that it made him close his eyes and take a huge swallow of beer. He opened one eye to see if Mickey had noticed, but the bartender was back at the other end of the bar, running his finger down an invoice, mouthing its contents to himself silently.

Why pick a familiar place? There was an entire city to choose from, a huge, teeming, concrete-and-glass ant-farm filled with strangers a hundred times removed. When he had finally admitted to himself just what he had to do, and how he would do it, why did the dart land directly on the square in his mind labeled "Mickey's Place"?

He needed to use the bathroom. His nervous system had been jangling like sleigh bells all the way, and another few minutes wouldn't matter anyway. When he stood up, he realized with a dull horror that he felt a little buzzed from the beers.

Should've eaten more dinner. He swung open the thin door of the men's room, walked in, then froze just inside. The front door had opened. Cautiously, he pushed the bathroom door open a few inches and peered out, craning his neck slightly to see over the jukebox that stood sentry between the men's and ladies' rooms like a gaudy old robot chaperone. Two young men, dressed to the nines, entered and strolled casually over to the middle of the bar.

Sal ducked back inside and began pacing back and forth the entire length of the bathroom, turning on a dime every five paces, the room being not much bigger than a large closet.

Sal's thoughts raced. The men were dressed to kill. That meant they'd been out. Late night business meeting, ending in a dinner? Movie? Opera? If they'd had dates, they brought them home before coming to the bar. That was good. Anyone dressed like that and coming into a place like this at such an hour on a weeknight must be looking for a quick nightcap, no more. Hopefully, they would toss one down and leave.

He continued pacing, the reason for his having gone into the bathroom in the first place now forgotten. He could wait it out. Those two fashion plates probably saw Mickey's as a place to slum, a little cave where they could soak up some local color, no more. They couldn't possibly imagine what a great place it was—He derailed that train of thought immediately. They'd be gone soon. Sal had noticed some coffee left over in the glass pot on the hot plate. It had probably been cooking there since Gettysburg, but it would help to clear his head and pass the time until the two strangers left.

The thought of that simple, plain, scratched coffee pot stopped him in his tracks. It was such an insignificant detail, yet, in the midst of the small tornado that had come to replace his rational thoughts, it made him smile right then and there. The very *familiarity* of it, that's what stopped him. A stupid coffee pot. But, everything about Mickey's Place was like that to him. He glanced up at the ceiling and traced with his eyes the familiar crack that ran across it from corner to corner, like a small dry riverbed. He must have looked up at that crack a couple of thousand times at least, as he did his business in there. He would have bet five thousand dollars easy that he could draw that crack perfectly on a piece of paper at home, every angle, every curve. That made him wince. Five thousand dollars? That was monopoly money now. His "creditors" would have probably cut him some slack, maybe even agreed to wait another week or two, for that kind of thin feed.

Sal resumed pacing, but very slowly now, his hands behind his back. Why pick Mickey's? Of all the places in this vast, anonymous city, why Mickey's? Why something so close to home, in more ways than one?

When the answer came, it was so obvious, there was no denying it. Because it's familiar. Exactly because it's so damn familiar! You can't betray a stranger. You can hurt a stranger, even ruin one, but you can only betray someone you really know. Sal knew the rhythms of Mickey's Place. He knew what Tuesday nights were like there. He knew how empty and desolate this part of town grew on weeknights. He knew that Mickey went to the bank every Wednesday, and that a strongbox hidden under a crate of empties contained a full week's haul. He also knew there was probably a car parked outside his apartment building this very minute, filled with people eager to bring his recent "business" transactions to a fruitful close. One way or another.

He knew he was wedged in nicely between a rock and a very hard place, and neither was going to give an inch. It was better just to act. No more nostalgia. No more philosophy. No more probing stares in the mirror. He turned, opened the door, and heard one of the strangers say too loudly, "Move it barkeep!"

Sal paused, edged his face around the doorframe, and peered above the jukebox. For a split-second, nothing registered; he felt like he was looking at a tableaux from a wax museum. Mickey was standing behind the bar, staring hard at the two fashion plates, who were standing directly across from him. One had both his hands on the edge of the bar, leaning in towards Mickey. The other was pointing a gun at Mickey's forehead.

"This isn't something you have to think about, my friend," said the first one.

"Give us whatever you've got besides the spare change in the register," added the one with the gun. He glanced at his wristwatch. "I can give you . . . let's see . . . fifteen seconds." Slowly, Mickey sank into a crouch, the first stranger leaning far over the bar to make sure the bartender didn't come up with anything more dangerous than cash.

Sal heard the sound of empty beer bottles clanking as Mickey pushed them aside to get to the strongbox. He ducked his head back just as the one with the gun darted a look around the bar. In the next second, Sal heeded his own counsel. No philosophy; no stares in the mirror. Crouching low, he pressed himself flat against the side of the massive jukebox, transferred the gun to his left hand, brought it around the side of the machine, peeked along its barrel and cried "freeze" in as threatening a tone as he could muster without any practice. The thieves whipped their heads around. The one with the gun pivoted, his eyes trying to focus on the exact spot from which the voice had come.

"God help me, I'll just start pumping this thing if you don't drop that gun. I don't care who gets hit!" Sal sounded frantic, which was good. Even if it hadn't been genuine, it was the right way to go. No one wants to deal with hysterics, especially hysterics backed up by firepower. The stranger dropped the gun and both men raised their hands over their heads.

"Kick it away from you. Over this way." The would-be thief did as he was told. Sal emerged from his improvised bunker, picked up the pistol and slid it down the bar towards Mickey, who snatched it up and trained it on the men.

"Call the police, Mickey. I'll watch these guys."

When Mickey neither turned towards the phone, nor said anything in reply, Sal glanced at him, keeping his gun trained on the strangers.

"It's okay, Mickey, I've got 'em. Call the cops."

To Sal's astonishment, Mickey waved the gun towards the front door and said only two words: "Get out." The men looked at each other with the same expression on their faces as the one on Sal, then they looked back warily at Mickey.

"Yeah, you heard right. You two bums get out. And God help you if I ever see you anywhere near this place again. Go on!" He punctuated those last words with another wave of the pistol. The men, still apprehensive, edged their way towards the door, looking back over their shoulders at Mickey and Sal. They opened the door and, convinced of their freedom, tore up the stairs without a backward glance. They pounded the pavement so hard in the desire to put distance between themselves and the bar, the sound of their heels smacking the sidewalk echoed in the still air for a few seconds.

Mickey lowered the gun and placed it on the bar. He looked at Sal with a curious, dull expression. It was sadness, plain and simple, and with a twist of disappointment added.

"Why did you let them go, Mickey? We had 'em dead to rights."

"Is that gun of yours registered, Sal?"

"Well, no, but . . . wait. You mean you didn't call the cops because of me?"

"Sit down here, Sal." As Sal perched himself on the familiar barstool, Mickey took two glasses and set them down on the bar. He poured three fingers of Jack Daniels into each. Then, he did something that Sal had never seen him do before, a small gesture, but one that would haunt him for years afterwards. Mickey didn't set the glass down in front of Sal, the way he'd been serving drinks to him for so many years now. Instead, he extended his index finger and placed it against one of the glasses. Then, he pushed the glass slowly until it was in front of Sal.

"How long have we known each other, Sal?" Mickey looked into his glass as he asked it.

"I don't know. Twenty years, maybe? Doesn't seem like it."

"I doubt you ever walked in here with a gun before, Sal."

Oh, God, no. Sal tried to read Mickey's thoughts, but the bartender—no, the friend—just kept looking into his glass, swirling the amber liquid around slowly.

"No, Mickey, you're right. I just needed some . . . protection lately. That's all."

"Mm-hmm," muttered Mickey, intent upon the little amber maelstrom in his glass. "Strange, you coming in here so late on a weeknight . . . on a *Tuesday* night, to boot . . . if it's so dangerous for you to be about. You see, it's not something you do, Sal. It's not *you*. And then, to walk in here with a gun in your pocket."

"What are you getting at, Mickey? Hey, if I didn't have that piece with me, those two guys would have robbed you, maybe shot you!" He tried to say it with hurtful pride.

When Mickey's eyes lifted from his glass, they were hard, serious. "You sat here all night like a zombie. You looked at me whenever I opened the cash register. You helped me get rid of old Franz. You jumped when Tom came up to you—yeah, I noticed. Then, you hung around until the place was deserted, fidgeting like a kid waitin' to talk to the principal. With a gun in your pocket, yet!"

"Now, Mickey . . ."

"Answer me, Sal. Answer me with the truth. Were you planning to rob me tonight?"

Sal contemplated lying, even contemplated laying the guilt on Mickey for suggesting such a thing. For one emotional, irrational second, the well-worn atmosphere of the bar seemed to envelope him like a blanket. Yeah, he knew Mickey and his ways, but Mickey knew him and his ways right back. The warmth of the place made him want to cry. How could anything rotten happen here? When he spoke, it was without philosophy, without nostalgia.

"Yes, Mickey. I was here to rob you tonight."

"Are things that bad?"

Sal only nodded, staring down at the bar.

"And what about afterwards? You couldn't have stayed around this town anymore, you know."

"I know that, Mickey. But, at least I would have been alive."

"Why me, Sal?"

Their eyes met. Sal bit his lip, the taste of whiskey in his mouth making it feel even drier.

"Talk, Sal. Why me?"

"Because . . . because you're my friend, Mickey." As bizarre as it sounded, for that one moment, the excuse sounded plausible to Sal, almost reasonable. People went to friends for help, when they were in trouble, right? He looked up hopefully into Mickey's face.

"I poured these drinks for a reason, Sal. This is one for the road. Drink up. It's the last one you'll ever have in here as long as I run the place."

"Mickey, please . . ." Sal wanted to plead, to make a case for himself, to bargain with Mickey, since things really worked out after all, what with the robbery attempt—*two robbery attempts*, he reminded himself—foiled. He wanted to say how even old friends can lose their minds sometimes and do really terrible things. But before he could utter another syllable, Mickey raised a hand to cut short anything else he might say.

"Sal, the only thing I wanna hear from you now is silence. The only thing I wanna see of you now is your back, as you walk up those stairs. I never wanna see the *front* of you again. That's one for the road, Sal. Drink up. It's closing time." Mickey turned, reached behind the cash register and snapped a light switch. The neon-lights in one of the front windows flickered, buzzed and died.

Sal downed the rest of his Jack Daniels, slid off the stool, and stopped with his hand on the doorknob, looking over his shoulder. Mickey rinsed off the two glasses, set them top down on a white cloth, and began wiping down the bar. He never looked up.

Outside, the early morning air was crisp. Sal stood for a few minutes at the top of the stairs, just looking up and down the dark street. In a clear sky shone a huge moon, so round it looked like it had been drawn with a protractor. It glowed with a mild, weary, buttermilk light. If you stuck arrows and numerals on its face, it could have been the twin sister of the clock hanging over the bar in Mickey's Place.

Sal crouched down and peered into the window of the bar. Mickey had set the chairs up on the tables and was sweeping the floor, shaking his head every once in a while. Sal turned, then, and started for home, wondering what more surprises might be ready to spring on him. Spring? Hey that's what traps do. Ha-ha!

The city was big, and generous in its own aloof way. If he somehow got through this night, the next day, the next week, there might be another Mickey's Place out there somewhere; a good, warm place where he would come to know the geography of the bathroom ceiling cracks like the lines of his hand, where the voices were always friendly. He'd have to start from scratch, of course, but it could happen. Maybe even before another twenty years had come and gone.

BIOGRAPHIES

Mark Alessio was born in 1955 in New York City. He studied English at New York University, then moved on to toil at various non-English–related jobs, including commercial air-conditioning repair and advertising market research. He has also performed in the United States and Europe as a guitarist in various Country music bands. Since 1996, his articles on religious topics have appeared regularly in the Catholic press. After spending one year in a Tibetan monastery, which he had mistaken for a very atmospheric Chinese restaurant, Mr. Alessio became a traditional Catholic. Today, he lives on Long Island, sharing a house with a refrigerator full of beer and some very bizarre memories. His brew of choice is Bass Ale.

Lucius Morris Beebe (1902–1966) was a personality of great renown, eventually appearing on the cover of *Life* magazine. He had the dubious distinction of being asked to leave both Yale and Harvard universities. In 1934, he began writing his column documenting New York cafe society called "This New York" for the *New York Herald*. A well-known bon vivant, Lucius was known for his acerbic wit, extravagant personal style, and gourmet taste, and was named one of the ten best-dressed men in America for several years. He wrote more than 30 books, many on the topic of railroading, one of his primary interests, as well as witty social commentary. Beebe was a prolific writer who wrote for many magazines such as *Holiday, Gourmet, Playboy, Newsweek,* and *Saturday*. In 1960, Beebe began writing a column called "This Wild West" for the *San Francisco Chronicle*, which continued until his death. This column is the source of his excerpts in this collection.

Hilaire Belloc (1870–1953) was in a village a dozen miles from Paris a few days before the start of the Franco-Prussian War. Because of the war, he and his sister were taken to England. He returned to France and then back to England, where he was educated at the Oratory School Birmingham, under Cardinal Newman, and later at Balliol College, Oxford. But before Balliol he went back to France to do his military service. He became president of the Oxford Union, but, probably because of his decided, and not always, fashionable views, failed to be elected a don after graduating. This remained a permanent disappointment and a grievance for him. His first book was published in 1896, and from then on he produced more than 150 volumes.

Martin Booe writes for the *Los Angeles Times* magazine, *Bon Appetit* and *Saveur,* and is coauthor of the cookbook *The Feast of the Five Senses* with Ludovic Lefebvre, chef of L'Orangerie in Los Angeles.

Ray Bradbury was born August 22, 1920 in Waukegan, Illinois. He graduated from Los Angeles High School in 1938, becoming a full-time writer in 1943. His reputation was established with the publication of *The Martian Chronicles* in 1950. Mr. Bradbury has written countless works since then, and is one of our greatest living writers.

Jean-Anselme Brillat-Savarin (1755–1826) is renowned as a lover of fine food and as the author of the *Physiologie de Gout.* A Royalist, he was in American exile during the French Revolution. Once back, he was appointed to various posts, finally becoming a judge on the Supreme Court of Appeal.

G. K. Chesterton (1874–1936) was born in London, England. A witty writer and convinced Catholic, he took on most of the great names in the literary world of his day. Along with his friend Hilaire Belloc and in books like the 1910 *What's Wrong with the World* he advocated a view called "Distributism," which is best summed up by his expression that every man ought to be allowed to own "three acres and a cow." During his life he published 69 books and at least another 10 have been published posthumously.

Colette (1873–1954), pen name of Sidonie-Gabrielle Colette. She belonged to the generation of authors that included Marcel Proust, Paul Valéry, André Gide, and Paul Claudel. Colette's career as a writer spanned from her early twenties to her mid-seventies. Her main themes were joys and pains of love and feminity in a male-dominated world. All her works are more or less autobiographical—Colette intentionally blurred the boundaries between fiction and fact in her life. She wrote more than 50 novels and scores of short stories.

Charles A. Coulombe (1960–20??), was born in New York City to an acting couple. Brought to Hollywood, California, at an early age by his parents, he and his family settled in the home of Criswell, the famed television psychic. An alumnus of New Mexico Military Institute in Roswell, he has written extensively on Catholicism, the Occult, Monarchy, Multi-Level Marketing, and other esoteric topics. *The Muse in the Bottle* is his first work on his favorite pastime.

Charles Cros (1842–1888), inventor of the gramaphone and precursor of color photography, was also a dedicated symbolist poet, and he knew such luminaries as Mallarmé, Rimbaud, and Verlaine.

Edward Davies was born in 1982 and educated at Carlton House Preparatory School and St. Edward's College, Liverpool, England. He has been a modern history undergraduate at Oriel College, Oxford, since matriculating as a member of Oxford University in October 2000. In September 2001 he was elected a Scholar by the provost and fellows of Oriel College, in recognition of his placement in the First Class after Honour Moderation Examinations. He is president of the Monarchist Society, treasurer of the Newman Society, and captain of the Oriel College Croquet Team.

Charles Dickens (1812–1870) was perhaps the most popular British writer of the nineteenth century. His literary reputation was made with *The Pickwick Papers,* from which his selection in the current work is taken. Such novels as *Oliver Twist, David Copperfield,* and *The Old Curiosity Shop* are rightly considered classics.

Andrew Dove is a pseudonym for a high-ranking officer within the U.S. military intelligence community. His name cannot be released due to the position of responsibility he holds and the sensitive nature of his work. Born in 1953 into a theatrical family in New York, he was relocated with his family to California at an early age. Dove was educated in the Catholic school system and was commissioned into the U.S. Army in 1978. During his military career, which has been spent primarily in the intelligence and special operations arena, he has held assignments as diverse as a special forces A Team commander, an intelligence officer for an SF company, a deputy director for intelligence at a special operations command, and a military advisor to the Peruvian Army Infantry School. Most recently he has been involved in counternarcotics operations, in particular, the war in Colombia. He makes his home with his wife of twenty-one years and numerous children.

Henry Fielding (1707–1754) was born at Wedmore, England. Between the ages of twenty-two and thirty, Henry managed to make quite a good living as a writer of farces and comedies for the London stage. He wrote several new plays a year, until the censorship laws hit in 1737 and closed down the playhouse he worked for. Deciding on a law career, Fielding entered the Middle Temple as a student in November 1737. He became a lawyer in 1740. In 1741, his first satirical novel, *Joseph Andrews,* appeared. Although his fiction brought him little money, his writings on law enforcement helped bring about the founding of the Bow Street Runners, London's first quasi-regular police force, and forerunner of Scotland Yard.

F. Scott Fitzgerald (1896–1940) was born in St. Paul, Minnesota, on September 24, 1896, the namesake and second cousin three times removed of the author of the National Anthem. Marrying Zelda Sayre, a Montgomery, Alabama, belle he had met during World War I, Fitzgerald and his wife became, both in his writing and their lives, the epitome of the Jazz Age. The excerpt here given is from a short story, "May Day," published in H. L. Mencken's magazine, *The Smart Set.* The unpleasant aftermaths of the Fitzgeralds' lives has done little to dull the alcoholic glamour conjured up by *This Side of Paradise* and *The Great Gatsby.*

Washington Irving (1783–1859) was born in New York City as the youngest of eleven children. In 1809 appeared Irving's comic history of the Dutch regime in New York, *A History of New York,* by the imaginary 'Dietrich Knickerbocker,' who was supposed to be an eccentric Dutch-American scholar. The name Knickerbocker was later used to identify the first American school of writers, the Knickerbocker Group, of which Irving was a leading figure. The book became part of New York folklore, and eventually the word Knickerbocker was also used to describe any New Yorker who could trace one's family to the original Dutch settlers. Irving's *Sketch Book* appeared in 1819–1820; it was a collection of stories that featured, in addition to the excerpt here, "The Legend of Sleepy Hollow" and "Rip Van Winkle," his most famous pieces.

Nicholas, Baron von Knupffer was born on August 5, 1976, into a noble Russian family known as "The Booze Barons of Willesden." He grew up without all the luxuries that great wealth and power could bring, but with all the joys of a good drink. His first experience of life was the exquisite taste of Veuve Cliquot seconds after birth, and life has only sweetened for him since.

Nora Lane is a poetess and screenwriter living in Los Angeles. Guarding her reputation, she refused to be named for this anthology, although she expressed "general solidarity with its purpose."

Jonathan Leaf is a writer living in Brooklyn, New York. He has written frequently for *National Review* and the *Weekly Standard*, among other publications. He is the author of an as yet unpublished novel about the 1960s, which critic Hilton Kramer said "seems to be a classic waiting to be recognized," and the forthcoming play "Pushkin," which critic James Wood called "a rare achievement in the modern age." He is a native of Trenton, New Jersey, and graduated from Yale.

H. P. Lovecraft (1890–1937) was born at his family home at 454 (then numbered 194) Angell Street in Providence, Rhode Island. "The Tomb," from whence the poem included here was taken, was written in the summer of 1917. His writing for such pulp magazines as *Weird Tales* eventually gained him posthumous fame as a master of horror fiction; this reputation was further buttressed by young writers such as August Derleth, Robert Bloch, and Fritz Leiber, whom he had encouraged and nurtured (the "Lovecraft Circle"). The poem here quoted is all the more remarkable, as H.P.L. was a life-long teetotaler.

Thom Loverro is a sports columnist for the *Washington Times*. He has been a journalist for twenty-five years, winning numerous local and national awards. He is also the author of three books, *The Washington Redskins: The Authorized History* (Taylor Publishing, 1996); *Home of the Game: The story of Camden Yards* (Taylor Publishing, 1999), and a biography on female hockey star Cammi Granato (Lerner Publishing, 2000). He is also a member of the adjunct faculty at the School of Communications at American University in Washington. Loverro lives in Columbia, Maryland, with his wife, Liz; two sons, Rocco and Nick; and his dog, Toby.

Arthur Machen (1863–1947) was born in Caerleon on Usk, in the county of Gwent, South Wales. Best known as a writer of such horror classics as *The Great God Pan,* he was also a social critic, with many affinities to G. K. Chesterton and Hilaire Belloc. As the essay republished here shows, he shared their views on alcohol.

John P. Marquand (1893–1960) was born on November 10, 1893, to Philip and Margaret Fuller Marquand, both descendants of old New England families. From 1915 to 1917, he was assistant magazine editor of the Boston *Transcript.* After a brief period as advertising copywriter in 1920 and 1921, he published *The Unspeakable Gentleman* (1922). Marquand was a frequent contributor of short stories to several popular magazines of the day. Many of his novels were also serialized in shortened form in these magazines. A recurring theme in many of Marquand's works concerns the life and times of the middle and upper classes in twentieth-century New England—particularly Boston—as illustrated in *The Late George Apley* (1937), *Wickford Point* (1939), and *H. M. Pulham, Esquire* (1941). He also wrote several mysteries featuring the Oriental detective Mr. Moto.

Lou Matthews is the author of *L.A. Breakdown,* named by the *Los Angeles Times* Book Review as one of the ten best novels of 1999. He was restaurant critic for *L.A. Style* magazine for 43 pounds.

Frank McCourt, although born in Brooklyn, came into public awareness in 1996 with the publication of his first book, *Angela's Ashes,* a highly colored memoir of his childhood in Ireland. After he returned to America in 1949, McCourt taught for thirty years in various New York City high schools and in city colleges. McCourt continued to explore his personal history with his second book, *'Tis: A Memoir,* published in September 1999.

H. L. Mencken (1880–1956) became, at the age of twenty-three, editor-at-large for the Baltimore *Herald.* In 1906, he joined the Baltimore *Sun,* writing and editing for the paper for much of the rest of his life. In 1917, Mencken was also relieved of his desk responsibilities, which freed him to write both for the paper, and also for his books and the magazines which bore his editing mark, *The American Mercury* and *The Smart Set.* His disdain for American society (he once described the States as "a

Commonwealth of third-rate minds") was doubtless in no small degree founded on Prohibition.

Ken O'Steen is a drinker and writer whose novels and essays have appeared in a number of guises in print and online, in America and in foreign realms. Born in North Carolina of Irish descent, he now lives and imbibes in Los Angeles, where he writes screenplays, when he is not doing a Balzac impersonation or exploring popular bars, where he is entirely unwelcome, patronizing haunts of little popularity where his presence is entirely appropriate. His main aspiration is to attain a state of bliss via numerous chemical agents.

Diana Paxson majored in English at Mills College and received an M.A. in comparative literature from the University of California. She is a writer of historical fantasy and lives in Berkeley, California, with her son, daughter-in-law, and grandchildren.

Titus Petronius Niger (??–A.D. 66), is best known as the author of the *Satyricon.* Seneca criticised him as a pleasure-seeker who "turned night into day." After his consulship, Petronius was made by Nero into his *arbiter elegantiae* ("director of elegance"), whose word on all matters of taste was law. Petronius was alleged to be involved with the conspiracy of Piso against Nero. Though innocent, he was arrested at Cumae in southern Italy. He did not wait for the inevitable sentence but committed suicide.

Craig Rice—Georgia Ann Randolph Craig (1908–1957), the subject of a recent biography by Jeffrey Marks (*Who Was That Lady*), was the creator of a number of memorable booze-soaked characters in just as booze-soaked mysteries. President Franklin Roosevelt (no stranger either to booze or mystery) confessed to being a fan of her work. As this excerpt from *8 Faces at 3* shows, she deserves to be better known.

C. E. Richard is a native Louisianian of Acadian French descent. He works as a writer and documentary filmmaker. His work includes a new book and a 6-episode series on the history of Louisiana. Both will be released next year in commemoration of the bicentennial of the Louisiana Purchase.

Jeremy Rosenberg lives in Los Angeles, California. He writes "The Secret City" column for latimes.com.

Spider Robinson was born in the United States in 1948. He moved to Canada in 1973. He has won the coveted Hugo Award three times. Mr. Robinson's Callahan stories have spawned quite an extensive cult following. They are comprised in the collections *Callahan's Crosstime Saloon* (from whence comes this selection), *Time Travelers Strictly Cash, Callahan's Secret, Callahan's Lady, Lady Slings the Booze, The Callahan Touch, Callahan's Legacy*, and *Callahan's Key*. He also has quite a few novels published.

Ruan Ji came from his native Henan province during the fourth century to be an official in the Wei capital of Loyang. Here he joined the Seven Sages of the Bamboo Grove. Well-known in China for his hatred of sanctimony, he drank in order to express his contempt for the corrupt officials of his day.

Thorne Smith (1893–1933) was born at the U.S. Naval Academy, Annapolis, Maryland. Known for a genial and comic treatment of supernatural themes, Smith's influence can be seen in many television shows (*Topper* and *Bewitched*), and movies (*Topper, Nightlife of the Gods, I Married a Witch*). A survivor of Prohibition, his attitude toward alcohol comes through clearly in his work.

Bert Randolph Sugar is a sports pundit, raconteur, and author of more than 50 books. He has founded two boxing magazines and appears frequently on television to discuss the sport, always clad in his trademark fedora and smoking a large cigar. Bert lives in Chappaqua, New York, and is currently writing a book on the Boston Red Sox–New York Yankees rivalry.

Mark Twain (1835–1910), pseudonym for Samuel Longhorn Clemens, is considered one of the greatest American writers. He is famous for *The Adventures of Huckleberry Finn* (1885), *The Adventures of Tom Sawyer* (1876), *A Connecticut Yankee in King Arthur's Court* (1889), along with stories, essays, articles, and much more.

Evelyn Waugh (1903–1968) wrote some of the most brilliant and bitingly satirical novels of his day. He converted to Catholicism in 1930. Later, as a reporter, he covered the Italo-Ethiopian War (1935–1936), an experience that was given fictional form in *Scoop* (1938). When World War II broke out, Waugh joined the Royal Marines and later the Royal Horse Guard, serving in North Africa, Crete, and Yugoslavia. Upon his discharge he retired to Somerset, which he made his home until his death. Sophisticated, caustic wit displayed in deceptively simple prose are the marks of such works as *Decline and Fall* (1928), *Vile Bodies* (1930), *Black Mischief* (1932), *A Handful of Dust* (1934), and *Put Out More Flags* (1942). His best-known works are *Brideshead Revisited* (1945) and the wartime trilogy made up of *Men at Arms* (1952), *Officers and Gentlemen* (1955), and *Unconditional Surrender* (1961). The Hollywood way of death is the subject of his only novel set in the United States, *The Loved One* (1948).